They Can Still Remember To Love

They Can Still Remember To Love

VICKI MIZEL

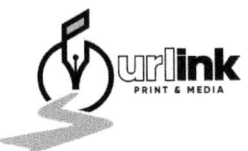

They Can Still Remember To Love

Copyright © 2021 by Vicki Mizel. All rights reserved.

No part of this publication may be reproduced, stored in a retrieval system or transmitted in any way by any means, electronic, mechanical, photocopy, recording or otherwise without the prior permission of the author except as provided by USA copyright law.

The opinions expressed by the author are not necessarily those of URLink Print and Media.

1603 Capitol Ave., Suite 310 Cheyenne, Wyoming USA 82001
1-888-980-6523 | admin@urlinkpublishing.com

URLink Print and Media is committed to excellence in the publishing industry.

Book design copyright © 2021 by URLink Print and Media. All rights reserved.

Published in the United States of America
ISBN 978-1-64753-623-7 (Paperback)
ISBN 978-1-64753-624-4 (Digital)

11.12.20

TRIBUTE

How Sasha my kitty inspired me to finally publish

Sasha is my gorgeous Seal Point Charcoal Snow Shoe kitty. She is beige with a black tail and nose, and four white paws. She has sapphire blue eyes and a little white chin. Years ago when she was a kitten, I took Sasha with me to my appointments. My physical therapist once told me she me she was the "Raquel Welch of cats."

Sasha also went to work with me when I was training to become a therapist. She helped me in the room with patients and was a healer too. Sasha was given to me when she was two months old. When I was trying to figure out a name for Sasha her beautiful blue eyes reminded me of a film producer I met in Russia in 1985. He had blue eyes. His name was Alexander but he was nicknamed Sasha. I loved the name and thus my baby girl became known as Sasha.

It was 2015 when I wrote this. I had lost my favorite job teaching acting. I'd had an abusive boss for years but I loved teaching the students so much and I belonged to the best set of teachers and artists, I had stayed until the district forced one thousand senior teachers out.

Then my two cats and I due to contamination had to leave our home and community; the neighbors and friends of 16 years at the Oakwood because of a combination of pesticide spraying in my apartment and ecoli in the next apartment. A pipe burst in the building and the water was filled with ecoli. There was an open dirt ditch that the manager refused to cover for months while the pipes were being fixed. The cats and I got so affected by vermin, debris and contamination, we moved off the grounds of Oakwood to another residential property.

The third apartment attracted flies and insects as it was too close to the trash dump.

Then we moved again only to the air of a constant smoking neighbor through the windows and balcony. We moved one more time and finally enjoyed our life for five years, until a renovation causing new problems. But I digress.

At Oakwood my cats could wander and enjoy the outdoors as I'd leave my door propped open when I was home. The kitties would greet the neighbors in the hallway, and roam down the stairs and take naps in the bushes. Now after this last move my poor kitties could no longer enjoy their (Indoor – Outdoor life).

They became Indoor kitties. They adjusted because our love was there and we were still all together. I think they felt sorrow as did I.

After that 5th move, I lost my energy at that point. I didn't realize how much the brain needs energy to function, to think, to dream, to envision, to believe and in making a thought into a reality, making something happen.

The afternoon sun shaded against the curtain as I lay in bed, my often daily ritual as I didn't have the energy yet to work. As I lay there I thought about my life. All the things I'd done. My happy childhood with Grandma Ida, Grandpa Harry, Uncle Bob, Aunt Flo, Uncle Morris, our dogs Sparky the beagle who taught me to walk. I practiced crawling with him all over the house and developed great motor skills.

We had two other dogs. Crystal our beautiful, white Samoyed we only had a short time and April the pretty female, all white with two brown spots on each hip, and a big tail who was the sweetest dog of all. She slept with me from the time I was 8 and a half until I was 24.

Jacqueline was my first kitty who was a Maine Coone. She was beautiful, smart and took walks with me. She lived to be 19 and a half.

I thought about all the wonderful things in my life. Acting, traveling, speaking and writing my book while getting my master's degree. Then I was hit by a big rig truck in an accident in January 1999 just 6 months before graduating. Yet, I still continued to finish and kept writing during and after the years of healing.

I acted in New York City on the stage. I experienced my dream of painting, dancing and finding myself teaching memory in Norway and in LA, San Diego and New York. I discovering my artistic self and then created and designed a program on career change named "Passion Quest."

I found out a decade later I received a 3.89 in my master's program. I could not believe I was that smart. That gave me confidence to move forward with my life. Then the best of all I finally in 2005 got my Dream Job I'd waited for my entire teacher career- teaching acting. Now that was gone. I was ill and didn't know how to have the energy to live. So maybe that was enough in a life. Maybe my best was behind me and there was nothing else to look forward to.

Sasha jumped onto the bed. Her slender body and beautiful tail sashayed as she moved closer to me. She was my constant comfort and love in my heart. She was the most important love connection in my life. (That's how I felt). Sasha crawled onto my chest her white paws on my heart. She looked at me, her blue eyes holding a steady contact as she downloaded her thoughts into me. "I am not going anywhere," she said. As if to mean to say that meant if I died she'd go through the rest of her days and nights without me, missing me. She needed IV fluids days due to the chemical pesticides, I couldn't leave her.

She is my "special person" and I am hers. When Sasha sleeps she will put her little white paw on my arm and nestle her head close to mine. I enjoyed having such a close, loving, furry companion.

Sasha looked at me in my "lost state." I felt her say, "Get your passion. Get your purpose again and make your life happen."

Then she held her gaze until she knew that I understood everything that she said to me. Once she felt it, that I got it; then she climbed off the bed and out of the room leaving me in my own space to think and digest what she just told me.

I lay back down in my bed looking up at the ceiling. My purpose? Where is my purpose? I decided to re-read my own book for myself. I needed guidance and I looked to that Dr. Vicki self to guide and empower my own self.

I read my book over a few days. Again lying in bed I thought, " I need to publish my book." I had already written it in 2006 and then with the difficulties of the abusive boss in 2007 all the way to 2013 and the emotional pain of rejection and his constant criticism, it was all I could do to hold on to the job.

That night I spoke with my spiritual teacher, Dr. Bruce Lane. We chatted.

He said, "You sound depressed."

I replied. "I am." I lost everything and I'm lost inside. I don't even know my purpose anymore."

He responded, "Yes, you know your purpose."

I said, "What is it?"

"You want to teach memory training to the whole world and you especially want to teach it to Alzheimer's and injured people to help them to know they can improve," he said.

"Oh yes that is what I thought I wanted to do but now I have no energy and I can't even remember things myself. " I answered.

I do not remember exactly what Dr. Lane said after that but I get the feeling that he shared that it was still my purpose and to "Ask the Light of the Most High to Guide me Back to Myself" and my life and health so I can continue to fulfill my dream. I think I was weary but relieved at the same time. I wasn't lost. I just had to get back on track.

As I continued to read my book the next afternoon, I realized in that moment if I died without publishing my book it would be a crime against humanity. I HAD TO PUBLISH MY BOOK!

Sasha walked in and climbed up onto the bed. Her gorgeous blue eyes softened as she looked at me. She came over and gave me a kiss with her beautiful face and little white spot on her chin. It was as if she was confirming, "Yes, this is the right decision for you."

Within about three days I received a call from Xlibris Publishing asking me if I was finally ready to publish my book. I told them, "Yes." It took 6 months and I did publish it. Then three weeks after publication I was hit in a hit and run on 1/1/16 as a pedestrian.

It has taken me this long to be well enough to try again. At this point I'm on my knees if God can make me well enough and help me with marketing and promoting the book I will publish again and I will make myself of service to train and teacher at least 3500 people/trainers in the world over the next decade. That is my mission.

I want to elevate the consciousness of all humanity that everyone can know the brain can regenerate and that Alzheimer's people can be improved. Even brain injured people can improve as I am a testament to this.

My heart aches as I write this. Sasha died July 3, 2019 at the age of 21.

It is her Spirit guiding me now to carry on and begin again.

Love,
Vicki

THEY CAN STILL REMEMBER TO LOVE

I dedicate this book to my Uncle Bob and Grandma Ida, for their love and continued beautiful memories they gave me that I carry with me. If it wasn't for them, I wouldn't have been motivated to have written this book. I wanted to help solve the problem of memory impairment. I don't want anyone to suffer as they did.

Love always and Happy Memories forever,

Vicki

CONTENTS

Acknowledgments 15
Introduction 19

PART 1

Chapter 1:   Uncle Bob in Early Stages and Getting Worse....... 25
Chapter 2:   They Can Still Remember to Love....................... 29
Chapter 3:   Personal Losses 35
Chapter 4:   My First Alzheimer's Speech, 1982 38
Chapter 5:   Bert and Selma 44
Chapter 6:   Viola and Lolly 50
Chapter 7:   All View.. 54
Chapter 8:   Philip 60
Chapter 9:   You Stir My Soul 68
Chapter 10: Insight into the Illness 72
Chapter 11: The Making of a Champion 79
Chapter 12: Wisdom of the Ages 86
Chapter 13: Awareness When Your Loved One Is Slipping 92
Chapter 14: Treatments for Loved Ones 96

PART 2

Chapter 15: Creating Your Life through Vision and
    Memory Methods..107
Chapter 16: Follow Your Dreams 127
Chapter 17: Passion Quest—Never Too Old 134
Chapter 18: If You Could Wave the Magic Wand—
    Creating Your Vision! 143
Conclusion 153

ACKNOWLEDGMENTS

For twenty-five years, I had desired to write a book. However, I didn't have the confidence or the trusted, directed, and loving guidance until I came to Holly Prado's writing workshops. I came to the class brain-injured and could only put a few words together. Through Holly's brilliance of encouragement and the compassionate, enthusiastic support of my classmates, I began roughly putting sentences together. It would take a month for me to write a full article. It took two and a half years of working with my seniors and coming home and "putting on the page," as Holly suggested, and bringing my material to class that allowed this book to unfold. What I didn't know is that what I was doing, no one else was. Not only that but I didn't know that I was getting responses, conversations, and improvements in my Alzheimer's patients that other people weren't getting.

When it came to editing, my class helped me rewrite each chapter at least eight times and then let me read aloud each work for an hour prior to each class for a year. To have the ongoing support for the decade this has taken is precious. I was treated kindly and respectfully even when I couldn't manage well because of other losses, tragedies, and injuries that occurred even after my traumatic brain injury. Imagine the "memory person" losing her memory. Yet a part of this book is how I gained it back through my work.

I thank Dr. Peter Whybrow and Dr. Andrew Leuchter. Both of these accomplished and world-renowned psychiatrists encouraged me to gain my master's degree and to write this book. For this, I am grateful that even when the "world" did not yet believe as I did, these two leading specialists in the field of psychology believed in my work and in me.

I want to also thank my brother, Gary. It was he who helped me see it through when I became brain-injured and didn't even have the ability to sooth myself when I was ill with a flu that chilled me to the bone. He stated, "You have only known treating people with memory techniques from a healthy brain. You will become a better healer and will have more empathy and understanding from experiencing an injured brain. That will help your future patients." He kept me encouraged through the years to keep my focus on completing the book.

I thank Peter Fischer, who believed this book would change the lives of those with Alzheimer's and create a new understanding for families, caregivers, and the medical professionals involved. Peter helped edit the book when he was in a nursing home later. He is now deceased, but I feel him each time I refocus on this work.

Special acknowledgments to Dr. Leonard Felder, Maureen Eagleton, Roderick Plummer, and Alice Shuman-Johnson for their constructive input and organization on content of the material. Additional thanks to Ben Bryant for his amazing eagle eyes on the technical edit.

I thank the twelve assisted living centers over the last twenty-five years that allowed me the chance to delve deeply and practice for many hours a week to discover and retest each theory and formulation on what can work with these patients or participants in both the Alzheimer's units and the regular assisted living for the "regular" seniors.

Praise goes to Dr. Dean Ortega St. John for being the first to hire me to give me a chance to find a way to heal Alzheimer's or improve the conditions by hiring me through the San Diego Community College. Dr. Ortega is still a dear friend and comrade twenty-five years later. Judy Canterbury was the nurse at the time in San Diego at one of the day care centers that noticed positive results of my work. She allowed us to film the Alzheimer's patients. Through this we proved that not only could they function and relate, but they could also have tremendous creative abilities for improvisation and pantomime. Judy too is still a dear friend whom I hope to work with and continue with her training others in this noted yet new field of healing potential of the brain.

I wish to thank Dr. Timothy Binder, Dr. Harold Toomin, as well as my many chiropractors, Dr. David Cauble, Dr. Leigh Tobias, a psychoanalyst who kept me steady throughout the ups and downs of practicing and publishing these works. I wish to thank my numerous massage therapists and healers to get me back into my own health and back to this business at hand of helping Alzheimer's patients and their families.

Special heart-felt acknowledgement goes out to Dr. Roger Bruce Lane, My Spiritual Teacher, for His Guidance and unconditional Love and Support.

I wish to thank all the doctors that met with me, disagreed with me, agreed with me, and recognized my deep passion for Alzheimer's patients and my desire to improve their lives, their families, and possibly stave off the illness in the future for genetic family members and the baby boomers of my generation.

I thank Voice America and Tacy Trump for my show, *Feeding Your Cells and Your Selves,* which enabled me to bring these twenty-five years of work and research to the forefront to a worldwide audience and show that this work is up to date with the "newest or latest" research.

Special thanks to my family members—my Uncle Bob and Grandma Ida—who, when they first became ill, still loved me so much. Writing this book was all I could do to try to first figure out how to help them and my other family relatives, such as Uncle Morris, in the future. Ultimately, through the first reading of this book, I realized, through my love and desire to "save" them, I am ultimately saving myself, my brain, my health, and my life. I wish for the readers to find the truth in these chapters and use what feels right for them to stave off these illnesses that can come from degeneration and old age. We have a chance for a bright future. However, we have to create it, plan it, nurture it, and make it happen. It doesn't happen by itself.

Ultimately, my thanks go to my Alzheimer's patients and the seniors I have worked with in both San Diego and Los Angeles. It is through them, our time together, our discovery together, our practice and my need for their love and their need to be needed and valued that this work was able to exist.

Thanks to my editor, agent, publisher, and to Dr. Eric R. Braverman for the introduction of this book.

INTRODUCTION

Eric Braverman, M.D.

When anyone hears a diagnosis of dementia, Alzheimer's, traumatic brain injury or stroke, it's alarming news. Such news is devastating to the patient's family, but mostly, to the patient. Without education about retraining the brain, feeding the brain, and stem cell treatments, one can only despair. A light goes out in one's life: "How long before I become impaired, so infirmed that I may not even know my name?"

This dilemma is now in the past. However, because of new technology in the last two years, there is more than just hope. There's a chance to regain abilities and, in some cases, even improve them.

In 1984, when medical science believed the brain could not regenerate, nor was there any help for Alzheimer's patients, Vicki Mizel was using memory training methods in the San Diego City Schools Unified District working with gifted students. At the same time, she became an advocate for her beloved uncle, who was suffering from Alzheimer's. In order for her to prove the validity of her memory system with Alzheimer's patients, Vicki was hired as a communications instructor at San Diego Community College, under the direction and guidance of Dr. Ortega St. John. She began working at two assisted living facilities and an Alzheimer's day care center.

Because of her efforts, group participants with Alzheimer's remembered positive, emotionally-packed events in their lives by recalling images of specific moments. Patients acted out their images in improvisational pantomime. Both patients and staff were thrilled.

Vicki then began a life-long study to help Alzheimer's patients, using her memory system. Some non-verbal patients started to talk. Some who were initially uninvolved would gradually become participants. Activity coordinators in various assisted living facilities noted that patients did not decline cognitively when Vicki was working with them.

What is remarkable about Vicki's research and the stories she shares in this book is that she discovered a connection between Alzheimer's and personal loss. Deep loss can mean loss of self. Vicki's work includes healing from grief, generating ways to create new passion, and purpose for oneself. This includes knowledge about good nutrition, exercise that promotes oxygen to the brain. Also, relationships with family and friends. Vicki's methods of exercising the brain can often help stave off further progression of memory impairment.

Only recently has medical science acknowledged that the brain can regenerate.

If society will reach out to memory experts like Vicki to train caregivers, medical staff and family members, there may be a decrease in mental deterioration in the elderly. Our aging population *can* remain active and healthy.

Our culture needs to be re-educated. If memory training became important in schools, children could get a strong cognitive beginning to help them learn and study throughout their lives. Memory training for baby boomers can strengthen their brains for the future. Memory training and stem cell treatments can restore those who have had head injuries and traumas. We no longer have to face the inevitability of cognitive decline. We have more opportunity for neural regeneration than ever before.

Stem cell treatments are becoming available. PATH Medical in New York, as of this year, offers such therapies and will be offering Vicki's memory training in the near future.

The personal stories and the specific guidance for memory improvement that Vicki Mizel presents in this fascinating book are not only worthwhile, but can be life restoring for any reader, of any age.

PART 1

CHAPTER 1

Uncle Bob in Early Stages and Getting Worse

Uncle Bob and I were driving in Los Angeles on one of my many trips to visit him. Uncle Bob was a handsome man, about five feet, eight inches tall. He had been a boy scout and had the body of a steady hiking master: slender, with strong legs and arms. His face was kind and sensitive, but today he was distressed. Uncle Bob knew the ramifications of Alzheimer's better than I did.

He said to me, "Listen, this is *very* important. In a couple of weeks, I may not know the location of the bank where I stored all the letters your mom sent me in my safe deposit box. We need to go to the bank and get them."

I said, "Okay, what's the name of the bank?" He shook his head. He couldn't remember. He had it written down. He pulled a paper from the side pocket of his shirt. I truly didn't believe that in a couple of weeks he'd forget. This was my own lack of understanding, not knowing what Alzheimer's disease really was.

He said, "Vicki, I drive down a street I've driven down for thirty-nine years, and now I can't find my way home. Nothing seems familiar." It was 1984; I was twenty-nine at the time.

I said, "Uncle Bob, you're probably just under stress with your job. High school students are difficult these days. I remember the stories you'd tell Mom. I really don't know how you could have stuck it out all these years. Plus, I know you're having trouble with your wife. She wants you back home. You've given in even though you really wanted to get a divorce. If you had kept your own apartment, become a writer and an artist, I don't think you'd be having so much anxiety right now."

I couldn't accept that my only living relative on my mother's side, my Uncle Bob, the scholar and creative writer, was losing his abilities. I couldn't cope with another loss.

I should have turned the steering wheel toward the bank and gotten my mom's letters, but I didn't believe him. I thought we had time. Those letters are lost forever, as are Uncle Bob's memories. He was trying in whatever moments he had of cognizance to complete what was precious in his life and pass it on to me.

When my Uncle Bob was placed in a nursing home, he was very sad and uncomfortable. He was desperate for help. He'd call me in San Diego, begging, "Help me! Help me! Get me outta here!"

Heartsick, I was allowed by his wife to take Uncle Bob for weekends, although it was a lot of driving. I'd pick him up in Los Angeles, drive him to my home in La Jolla for us to enjoy a few days together, and then I drove him back. He couldn't take a train or bus by himself.

One particular time, I took Uncle Bob to Seaport Village in San Diego, California. They have a carousel. Uncle Bob reminded me that when I was three years old, my mom, dad, Grandma Ida, Grandpa Harry, and he would let me ride the carousel over and over at Disneyland. I loved the horses going up and down and spinning around so I could take in the view as we circled. "Remember that?" We reminisced. Uncle Bob said to me while we were on the wooden horses, "In little moments like this, I feel such happiness." He had a tear in one eye; he must have wiped the other tear from his cheek. Just like a man, he said the sun had got in his eyes, causing the tear.

After our ride on the carousel, we sat down for some lunch, and I showed him a pad of cartoons. Uncle Bob was a good artist. He'd draw little cartoons on a pad of paper and then flip them, making them come to life. He took out his pencil. I gave him a blank pad. Within ten minutes, he gave it back to me. He had drawn little pictures for me to make a moving cartoon. "You can still do that! Wow, Uncle Bob, that's great!"

He'd tire easily after a few hours, so we'd go home to rest. He had to take his insulin shot for his diabetes. He still knew how to do that.

He also wanted to go to the Wild Animal Park. The next day, he was up and dressed at 6:00 a.m. The park didn't open 'til 10:00 a.m. He came into my room. "I'm ready," he said.

"Oh, Uncle Bob," I moaned at the hour. "We can't leave yet. The park doesn't open for a few more hours." He just couldn't wait.

What I remember most about that day is that he smiled the whole time. He felt comfort in my presence. We were part of our original family—that connection remained whether or not the ability to function on a day-to-day basis did. He told me how happy he was for us to be together. "I have freedom like a bird," he said, "to be out of my nursing home prison."

Sometimes I'd just come to LA and take him out to Nate and Al's for our favorite beef brisket and potato pancakes. Uncle Bob and I used to play talking to each other in accents. He was good at drama, as was I. I inherited it from him and my mom. Even in his last days, if I spoke to him as a Brit, he'd answer me in a British accent. If I spoke in New York or Russian accents, he always matched me in that accent.

Once at the nursing home, the nurse began to undress him in my presence. He felt uncomfortable, so I walked out of the room. The nurse said to me, "Oh, he's not aware." How could they not notice his expression of fright and embarrassment for his niece to see him that way? I could see this maybe because I knew him. We had a connection, a strong bond invisible to the eye, but it held us together. I had that with my Grandma Ida too.

I had accepted what had become his limitations. Our love was still limitless, present beyond other capacities no longer in our control. I understand this illness much more now, twenty-six years later. Perhaps this is why it's easy for me to see real people when I walk into a room of Alzheimer's patients. I see their eyes, their hearts, and their spirits.

CHAPTER 2

They Can Still Remember to Love

Remarkably, medical science had always said the brain could not regenerate. As recently as 1990, top medical doctors and scientists concluded that unlike the skin, hair, nails, and human tissue, the brain, after its full development by the age of twenty-five, ceases to grow new cells.

My experience as a memory teacher and a communications instructor led me to think differently. In 1984, I spent three months attempting to have my Alzheimer's group from the Alzheimer's Day Care Center in San Diego, California, memorize a list of items. This is the first step in learning how to associate information. They'd remember a list for five minutes (after many reviews and much prompting), but two days later, 90 percent of them drew a blank. I'd reintroduce the association method and explain how the brain worked, but still nothing.

Then I asked them to tell me about one of the most important or special days in their lives. Each person answered that it was his or her wedding day. I had each person share that special day with me and describe what he or she remembered most about it. Then we'd focus on one particular tangible image to be their symbol of that day. For Margarette, a charming Hispanic woman, it was the kiss. Bert, a German gentleman, remembered the opera house in Minsk. Gus, a native of California, recalled the organ grinder with the monkey. For Charles from Oklahoma, it was his pig, the family pet that went everywhere, even to weddings.

Finally, Steve, a native of San Diego, remembered golf clubs; he and his wife spent their honeymoon golfing.

I hired an artist to draw pictures of the kiss, the opera house, the organ, the pig, and golf clubs. The next week, I pointed to the pictures and asked the group, "Who was the kiss?" Margarette raised her hand and said, "That's me." I asked, "Who was the organ?" Gus waved his hand. As I went around the circle, each person remembered his or her symbol from the wedding day. This was a groundbreaking observation. Even after a week, with a picture cue, they remembered. This reinforces the idea that short-term memory can become long-term memory by making a tangible picture.

At that time, Dr. Carl Sagan, the noted scientist, had presented a television special discussing the inner space of the mind called *New Frontiers of the Mind*. I liked him, what he'd said, and thus felt drawn to read his book, *Dragons of Eden*.

In chapter 2, page 46 of *Dragons of Eden*, Dr. Carl Sagan clearly explained the notion of neural branch growth in the brain. This was written in 1977: "A remarkable series of experiments on brain changes during learning has been performed by the American psychologist Mark Rosenzweig and his colleagues at the University of California at Berkeley. They maintained two different populations of laboratory rats—one in a dull, repetitive, impoverished environment; the other in a variegated, lively, enriched environment. The latter group displayed a striking increase in the mass and thickness of the cerebral cortex, as well as accompanying changes in brain chemistry. These increases occurred in mature as well as in young animals. Such experiments demonstrate that physiological changes accompany intellectual experience and show how plasticity can be controlled automatically. Since a more massive cerebral cortex may make future learning easier, the importance of enriched environments in childhood is clearly drawn."

"This would mean that new learning corresponds to the generation of new synapses or the activation of moribund old ones, and some preliminary evidence consistent with this view has been obtained by the American neuroanatomist William Greenough of the University of Illinois and his co-workers. They have found that after several weeks of learning new tasks in laboratory contexts, rats develop the kind of new neural branches in their cortices that form synapses. Other rats, handled similarly but given no comparable education, exhibit no such neuron-anatomical novelties. The construction of new synapses requires the synthesis of protein and RNA molecules. There is a great deal of evidence showing that these molecules are produced in the brain during learning, and some scientists have suggested that the learning is contained within brain proteins or RNA. But it seems more likely that the new information is contained in the neurons, which are in turn constructed of proteins and RNA."

From reading this, it became clear to me that Dr. Sagan was discussing how the synapses of the brain formed an architectural scaffold. The idea of synaptic firing causing neuro brain growth became my new belief, even though the "doctors" of the time didn't want to believe a twenty-five-year-old teacher. Still, I quietly continued.

As I was having these positive experiences with my Alzheimer's patients, witnessing their memories growing, I sought out a medical specialist in memory at the University of California at San Diego. The late Dr. Nelson Butters, the MD, PhD who ran the Psychology Department at UCSD and had worked for thirty years with memory problems involved in Korsakov syndrome, viewed a video of mine as I worked with the Alzheimer's patients. He wrote in a letter to me, saying: "I didn't know this kind of creativity still existed in these patients." Yet, according to the rest of the world at that time, my findings were premature: I was not a doctor; mine was only a narrative accounting. There was no equipment yet sensitive enough, such as SPECT and PET brain imaging, to measure these obvious objective findings in the brain.

The Berkeley rat experiments were not getting the publicity that the same study received twenty years later.

Now, some of those same medical doctors and medical scientists are refuting their earlier works, agreeing with the neurogenesis theory that the brain can regenerate. Dr. Gary Small, author of *The Memory Bible*, also concurs with the neural sprouting concept. He wrote: "Thanks to UCLA and others, we now have the stunning breakthrough discovery of PET scanning and finally see this kind of subtle brain dysfunction in living humans." (Prior to this, it could only be seen in autopsy.)

Memory enhancement programs have mushroomed now for older adults. In schools, research is providing evidence that the more a child's mind is stimulated, the more the dendrites in his or her brain can grow. Neural sprouting is possible in the child, the baby boomer, and the senior—in any one who continues to stimulate and enhance learning.

We know through this medical research that the brain can regenerate, which leads me to the central concern of this book. Officially, no one knows what causes Alzheimer's disease; however, my experience over the past twenty-five years indicates that in a majority of Alzheimer's patients, there is a significant emotional loss prior to the onset of the physical illness. It is a loss that affects emotional well-being, whether it is loss of a job, loss of a mate, depression, unprocessed grief, or leading a life no longer enjoyable over a period of time. Depletion then affects the mind, i.e. brain chemistry, physically. With the help of medical brain applications such as those developed by Dr. Daniel Amen in Newport Beach, California, and Dr. Michael Usler at the UCLA Brain Clinic in Santa Monica, we can more accurately measure microscopic and molecular brain functions. Regarding the changes occurring today in many baby boomers, Dr. Gary Small states in his book *The Memory Bible* on page 22, "These tools may also help us to gauge the success of memory fitness programs and other interventions at slowing the brain aging process down."

And so the information in these pages of my book, *They Can Still Remember to Love*, is scientifically accurate, dovetailing with all the research of top scientists and doctors of our time. The idea of new neural sprouts, which I coined "brainsprouts," is alive and available for us all.

Yet, even with this new awareness, as recently as March 6, 2006, in an Alzheimer's segment on a national television channel, it was stated: "There is nothing we can do about Alzheimer's." I disagree. It has been my experience that the combination of recreating a new passion and purpose in our senior years can excite the mind.

Regaining oneself after a significant loss—be it a mate, a career, one's health or a life previously known—takes great effort. Support is necessary to help pull together the parts of a self again. Without this support, one often continues to live an unsatisfying life or is too focused on the past not on the present.

With my own peers or with seniors I know of, often the feeling is that "I'm too old to change. I'm too old to bother." Yet, as the baby boomers become a multitude of seniors and most likely centenarians, this generation will have to continue to grow, to learn, to adapt, and to change.

With that will come a new form of aging, a new attitude toward aging. Our country cannot afford to have the majority of Americans in nursing homes, shuffling around in walkers or sitting in wheelchairs. This would debilitate our country and our resources. It is up to us to recognize that there is no retirement from living, from taking care of our mental, emotional, and physical health. It is our responsibility to change, and, with that, change society's view of aging and the aged. We can continue to be strong. This book takes the time to explore these possibilities and theories on all levels.

Sadly, I was not able to save my Uncle Bob. He died of pneumonia in the nursing home. But I hope this work, which I began because of him, can help families, caregivers, spouses, and Alzheimer's patients themselves. I hold a master's degree in psychology from Antioch University and have had seven years of training as a psychotherapist. I have worked with hundreds of seniors and Alzheimer's patients. I hold a secondary teaching credential in speech communication, a community college teaching credential in psychology, and a California lifetime teaching credential.

My mother said that success is this: Making the world a better place to live. My original idea in helping Alzheimer's patients was to keep those I loved alive. Now, it is important to me that all of us keep our loved ones and ourselves alive and mentally available.

CHAPTER 3

Personal Losses

Some people thought it was unusual for a twenty-five-year-old woman to want to spend time with Alzheimer's patients instead of being out, dating, and doing things young people did. I was asked how I became interested in Alzheimer's disease. My answer was simple: "need." When I was twenty-two, my mother passed away at the very young age of fifty-two. I became estranged from my father when he remarried and moved away from La Jolla, California, to Albuquerque, New Mexico, despite my desire to stay close. I met a nice man shortly after he had finished law school. We dated a few months, and then he too moved away. I didn't know how to deal with so many losses at once. No one else in my group of friends had lost parents and grandparents or a lover.

Every day, I woke up in tears. I knew I had to work through this. I was young. I had a full life ahead of me. Then I thought, "What do people do who have had losses like this or have lost mates after forty, fifty, and sixty years? Do they shrivel up and die, or do they still create a future for themselves?"

Grief is a tough emotion. It's unpredictable. One never knows when it's coming. Tears fall. Does one sleep too much or too little? Reminiscing becomes the present tense because the pain of the present without the loved one is just too much to bear. I had thought this kind of pain was only for an old person. Then it hit me. Maybe this is a form of what Alzheimer's patients experience in the first stages of losing a mate. I thought about my grandmother.

After the death of my grandfather, she began having memory loss and confusion. I tried to go back in my mind, analyze what she must have been feeling. First, the pain hurts so much that one tries to forget. Then, the forgetting becomes depression. Depression over an extended period of time can cause memory loss. There is a tendency to think backward instead of forward, creating future goals. I wondered if one could actively work through grief, then find new goals with passion and purpose. If so, perhaps this could offset the pattern that many widows and widowers fall into. I was hoping that from my suffering and grief at a young age, I could help Alzheimer's patients. Could I give them renewed life?

I found that my grief lessened. Maybe my memory system could help seniors or even early-stage Alzheimer's patients. This brings up the question of whether one aspect of Alzheimer's could be caused by emotional grief. Could chemicals in the brain be changed enough to cause or contribute to cell death? I knew there were many medical reasons for cell death: lack of oxygen to the brain; genetics; abnormal proteins, which can be caused by malabsorbed nutrients that do not allow the RNA and DNA to be properly duplicated in the cell. The fourth cause is attributed to cells contaminated by pollutants in our air, food, and water. We know Alzheimer's is a form of cell strangulation by hardened protein tangles that keep the cells from breathing. Other cell deaths can result in forms of dementia. But no one in my research had suggested any emotional causation. My curiosity increased.

How do older adults handle loss? I remember speaking to Holocaust survivors. Some were people I met in the nursing homes; others were parents of friends of mine in Los Angeles. I asked what kept them going. Victor Frankl wrote an entire book, *Man's Search for Meaning*, on this question. He states that what keeps the will going are vision and purpose. One lady I interviewed said she got through her time in a concentration camp because she lived for the taste of chocolate and to see Hitler go down. Another woman said that she lived to bear a son in America who could be a college graduate and become an attorney. Yet another Holocaust survivor found a thousand dollars on a dead man and took a chance escaping into the forest. All these people had vision and hope.

CHAPTER 4

My First Alzheimer's Speech, 1982

Although I was sure that my memory system could help Alzheimer's patients; I hadn't enough evidence.

I was giving a speech at my Toastmasters group in La Jolla California in 1982. I was discussing the topic of memory training and how it improved brain function. I had expressed a desire to work with Alzheimer's patients because of my uncle's memory problems. One of the ladies at my Toastmasters group, Charlene, said she worked in a nursing home in Mission Hills. Would I like to come teach some of my memory techniques to her students? I was thrilled at such an opportunity.

We set up a time, and I went for about an hour. The group was in a living room area of a small home in the Mission Hills area of San Diego. The audience was seated on brown chairs and a couch with a flowered pattern on it. There were floor lamps and table lamps resting on the end tables next to the chairs. I asked the group to look around and notice items in the living room where we were sitting. We'd create a list together. The list was "chair, plant, and lamp." One man remembered "chair" and "plant," because he used to water a plant for his wife every day. He also remembered "lamp." But it wasn't a lamp in the room; it was the memory of a lamp in his first home, over fifty years ago. He remembered that lamp in his mind's eye, although he couldn't make out the lamp directly in front of him.

To memorize the list, I had the group envision steps using their imagination and connecting the words in a visual, unusual way, with the items in motion: the chair was dancing with the plant, and the plant was turning on a lamp. After the group tried to memorize the list, we chatted and told stories. At the end, Charlene, my friend, asked the group what was on the list.

They remembered the items. Charlene was amazed. She told me that they never remember, especially the last item, after another activity like our story telling. The reason they remembered is because when we make connections between two items in motion with an unusual association, it changes the way the information is encoded into our mind. The mind sees pictures rather than words. This changes what would have been short term memory into long term recall.

In graduate school in 1980, before I dropped out to begin my memory business, I learned of a term called "retroactive inhibition." Usually, the mind only remembers the last thing it learns. However, when information is stored into long-term memory, one can remember a sequence at any point, not just the last thing learned. I did my first study on that. I had people remember a list. Then I taught them the method of association and then told a joke after they memorized the list, using this brainsprouts memory method. Everyone who used the method properly could still remember the list. This is why even the Alzheimer's patients could recall the items.

Charlene, too, was now even more curious. She asked if I could address a larger audience, give a speech at their clubhouse to a group of seniors and Alzheimer's patients at one of their monthly get-togethers. I happily agreed.

It was a Tuesday evening. I was worried about looking old enough to have credibility. I was twenty-six at the time. I wore a blue pin-striped suit that I had purchased at Nordstrom for $400.00. I had never spent that much money on clothing before that time. I felt that was how I needed to dress to allow my audience to feel safe enough to hear my words. I had never talked to a large group of Alzheimer's people. I walked down a few stairs into a clubhouse. I thought it looked like the den of an old country club with a moose head hanging on the wall. The floors were wooden, but once I saw a chalkboard, being a teacher, I felt comfortable. There were about fifty people.

So, I began to speak about memory. I drew little pictures on the board. I discussed short-term and long-term memory. Then I gave an analogy: the memory system is stimulating to the mind as if the mind were a tree; this memory system stimulates new growth like new tree branches. I said the memory system adds stimulation the way nutrients for a tree could increase the trees capacity to make new foliage, sprout leaves, and bear fruits. I explained Alzheimer's disease as if neurons were a squirrel, but it was a tired squirrel unable to jump from one tree branch to the other. I was trying to speak in a way they could understand. I didn't think that if I said the neurons couldn't fire from the synapse into the sodium pump, it would make much sense to them.

I was very direct about the illness. They all listened and yelled out from the audience. One man said, "What if the tree is near a telephone wire, and then there is a lightning bolt and it strikes the tree?" I looked at him with some surprise and quickly thought how to incorporate it into my speech. I said, "It would injure the tree and its branches, which is very much what Alzheimer's or a stroke can do. It can injure the brain, which is like our tree." The man said, "What if lighting strikes it again?" I felt challenged.

I recalled a woman I had worked with named Signa. She had a stroke. She got much better very quickly—within a few weeks—by incorporating the memory system into her physical therapy. I explained to Signa that the stroke to her brain is analogous to a tree getting injured by lightning striking it. Over time, the tree will have new foliage and growth in the springtime, much as the associations we were making in our sessions stimulated new neural connections in her brain. We began with simple memory associations. She imagined her daughter coming to the hospital to hug her. Then we had her daughter read to her from a letter. Then we had the letter open the window and smell the fresh air. It seemed like such a small activity. Within three weeks, just five to ten minutes a day of making simple picture associations and connecting them worked. Both the physical therapist and speech therapist came to me and said to me, "Whatever you're doing with her, it is working. She's improving much faster than we had anticipated." The next time I saw Signa I told her how pleased everyone was with her rapid improvement. Then, I said, "In fact, I bet you'll get to go home soon."

She stopped improving. She didn't want any more memory lessons. What I hadn't known was that she was under tremendous stress at home, which is what had caused the stroke in the first place. Why should she continue to get better if she was going back to the same place that caused the injury in the first place? That taught me something. You have to fix the problem, then provide the follow-up care and support in goal planning.

I answered the man's question. "Well, if we moved the tree, it would be disastrous for the tree. It would be uprooted, which would be too stressful. The tree couldn't grow. So, we'll have to move the electric wire to another location. Then the lightning is less likely to strike the tree again." I felt the audience agreeing with me. They had gotten to a place where they were under some kind of stress, internal or external, and it made their memories shut down.

One man raised his hand. "I was a helicopter pilot. I flew everywhere in fighter and commercial planes. Then, they retired me." That was it. Basically, he had stopped living because he no longer felt valuable or important.

Another woman said she had worked for Disney on *Snow White*. She said Disney was like a family then. Walt was a fine man. She said they had drawn each celluloid image for the movie, frame by frame. It took six months just to get one full scene of Snow White with the dwarfs. "Did you know you were creating a hit that would go down in history?" I asked. She smiled. "We had no idea. We just knew we loved the work, and we enjoyed working with each other." How could this woman of so much talent with such a history now be spending her days in a nursing home unable to walk, losing a grasp on reality?

The cells in the skin regenerate. We have reparative qualities in our bodies for illnesses, accidents, and injuries. There must be a way for the brain to regenerate. I felt firmly that my memory system did indeed assist regenerative qualities in the brain from existing living cells.

Until we can measure the brain microscopically, it is difficult to see these cells multiply. But stimulation can be seen from CAT and PET scans in a living person. I imagine our brain stimulated by the chemical electrical recall of "re-seeing" pictures in our mind. Perhaps this produces "heat" in the brain, thus creating new neural branches from the existing live cells. This is just an analogy, although it would be amazing to be able to measure the microscopic activity in the brain neurons while practicing the memory system of recall.

Unfortunately, most research on the human brain is done by autopsy.

As I was continuing my speech, one person yelled out, "What about names? How do we remember names?" I asked the lady in the front row what her name was; she said it was Elizabeth. I explained when you remember a person's name, you break the word into syllables, then you make each syllable into a tangible picture. I said, "With Elizabeth we have E Liza Beth—four syllables. E Liz A Beth." One gentleman yelled out, "A Tin Lizzie." I didn't know what that was. They explained to me it was the Model T Ford. I was thrilled.

The group was with me, I was learning from them. I explained that they could imagine the Tin Lizzie falling into a bathtub. They could look also for an outstanding characteristic on the person's face, Elizabeth, and then associate the picture. Elizabeth thought her curly hair was her outstanding characteristic. We made a visual picture of her getting into the Tin Lizzie and driving with her hair blowing in the wind. Then, the car smashes into a full bathtub. The group laughed, but they did remember her name.

That night, my heart became involved, and my heart, to this day, never has wavered. The memory system can help those who have been given up for lost.

CHAPTER 5

Bert and Selma

One of the problems with Alzheimer's patients is they cannot cue themselves. They must depend on an outside object as a cue, thus triggering an image. Also, because of the impairment to the brain, images have a difficult time sticking in the mind. However, employing the method of imagery, then enhancing the image by using all of the senses, information is anchored so that it can be recalled, once cued.

Bert, a German gentleman, was at the Alzheimer's Day Care Center in San Diego, California, where I worked. Every day, at least twenty-five times an hour, he would very politely, in his charming foreign accent, get up and call to the nurse, "Excuse me, lovely miss, tell me please, when is my wife coming to pick me up?" He would ask this as if he had never asked the question before. The nurse would look at him and say, "Four-thirty. Your wife is coming to pick you up at four-thirty."

Bert would slowly walk back to his chair, sit for a few minutes, then get up and walk over to the nurse again and say, "Excuse me, lovely miss, tell me please, when is my wife coming to pick me up?" This went on day in, day out. I learned of this and went over to work with Bert to see if by making the information into pictures and linking the information I could help his retention. I said, "Bert, can you imagine seeing a great big clock in your mind?" I pointed to the clock on the wall. "Imagine this four times as big." Bert had lived in Minsk, Bella Russe, and in the town square, there was a large clock. He could imagine this in his mind. "Yes," he answered.

"Bert, I want you to imagine you are taking your right hand. You are turning the hands of the clock, so the clock would read 'four-thirty.' Can you imagine seeing that?"

"Yes," he said proudly.

"Next, I want you to see yourself embracing your wife and kissing her hello."

"That I can see. I love my wife. I hug my wife, and she smells so nice."

"Next, I want you to see your wife taking you to the car then opening the car door. I want you to imagine the feeling of getting into the seat of the car and the car door closing." I repeated these visuals along with the connections a few times: Bert sees himself turning the hands of the clock; the clock hugs his wife. (He is personified as the clock.) His wife opens the car door. Bert gets in. It worked! Bert was able to link the images. After that, he used to say to the nurses, "You want to meet my wife, she'll be here today at four-thirty."

By using these images and embellishing them, accessing the information as well as using the senses—hugging, seeing, smelling, kissing, hellos—all these enhance the ability to anchor memory in the brain. This helps the Alzheimer's patient lock into the picture and thus recall more often than without employing these techniques. Consequently, communication becomes less frustrating for caregivers and family members.

This was in San Diego in the 1980s. In the 1990s, I was in NYC acting and in LA working on my master's degree in psychology. After my car accident in 1999, I needed a way to get my own memory back. So I decided that after graduating in 2000 from Antioch University, I'd return to teaching my Alzheimer's seniors in LA. This might help me regain my own memory.

Jewish Home for the Aged was the first site where I worked as an adult school teacher for Reseda, California. I began in July 2001. Although I had worked with the Alzheimer's patients in San Diego from 1984 through 1989, I had been away from memory training; I wanted to see if my theories held true almost fifteen years later. I went three days a week, working with different groups. After a year, I was feeling very connected to one particular group.

"Can you help Selma?" Gina, the activities director, asked me. Gina was a kindly middle-aged woman. Selma was in her eighties with white hair, smooth skin, a white puffy face, and pretty blue eyes.

"I'm scared. I am frightened." Selma was shaking. I turned to Selma and sat down next to her. I took her hand.

"I'm here, Selma." She seemed relieved to see me and grabbed my hand a little tighter. I said, "Let's breathe."

Together we took three deep breaths. "Remember to breathe, Selma, when you feel nervous."

"I am scared and nervous." She was going back into her shaking mode.

"Where would you feel safe?"

"In my home."

"Where is your home?"

"That's what I don't know. That's why I am scared. I don't remember."

I wheeled Selma to her room in her wheelchair. She's wasn't really crippled, but her feet were puffy. She has a debilitating medical condition. I showed her where her room was and then had her touch her bedspread.

"What does it feel like, Selma?"

"It's rough."

"What color is it?"

"It's purple." (It was pink, but close enough.) Then, she said, "I remember this moment, but in five minutes, I won't remember."

"That's okay."

"No, it's not okay. That's what's so upsetting. I can't remember anything."

"Do you remember me?"
"Yes, because you're here."
"You remember your son."
"I don't see him so much."
"But you remember him. So, it's true. You do remember some things? Right?"
"Yes, but I can't remember anything."
"Selma, you remember me."
"I can remember some things. I can remember some things, okay."

I asked her, "Can we go to the birthday party? Let's go. If you don't want to stay, we'll leave." She agreed.

There is a monthly celebration for all those residents who have a birthday. Everyone joins together in the dining room. There is live entertainment, musicians who play wonderful old tunes for at least sixty people who were singing and laughing.

When we got to the party in the large eating area, fresh fruit salad was being served with cake and ice cream. The fruit salad was some of the best I had ever tasted, but Selma didn't want any. She just couldn't relax, couldn't enjoy herself.

"I want to go back."
"You don't want to enjoy the music, Selma?"
"No, I want to go back to my home."

I finished my last bite of fruit salad and came around to unlock her wheelchair. I began to wheel her chair forward. Gina saw us leaving and said, "Oh, Selma, aren't you enjoying the party?" She spoke with a concerned, loving voice.

"No, it's too much for me!"
"Selma, watch as we go back. I'll show you landmarks so you don't have to be so afraid. You'll know how to get back to your room yourself," I said.
"No."
"No?"
"No, I can't. I can't remember."
"But, Selma, you remember me and your son."
"It's too hard. I don't want to try."

"What would happen if you tried?"

"I'd fail."

"So, you don't want to try to remember anything at all because of the fear of failing."

"That's right."

"So, the feeling of failing is too uncomfortable for you?"

"Yes, that's right."

"Selma, was there a time when you could remember?"

"Yes, when I was a teenager and I didn't have any responsibilities so everything was easy to remember. It was fun and easy."

"Selma, you don't have any responsibilities now. Everything here in the home is done for you."

"Well, I don't know."

I said, "Selma, I have a thought, and I want your feedback on it."

"Okay."

"I've never been married, and I am forty-seven. Now, I can approach this two ways. I could say, I'll never ever get married since it hasn't happened to me."

Selma states, "You've closed your mind. If you close your mind, then you'll never have that opportunity available to you."

"That's a good point, Selma."

"Or I could say, up until now, I haven't met the right person to marry, but it could happen. I am open to meeting my husband."

"Well, it's up to you," Selma said, looking straight at me.

"Selma, it's the same for you. If you close your mind then you don't have a chance to remember, even if you want to."

"I have closed my mind, and I've lost the key."

"You've lost the key?"

"Yes, I don't know where it is."

"Selma, who has the key to your mind?"

"I don't know. I don't know. Maybe I do."

"Yes, I think so."

"I have the key to my mind."

This entire conversation was taking place while I was wheeling Selma back toward her room. We stopped by the nurse's station just before her room and continued our conversation. We were facing each other.

"Yes, Selma, if you want you can open it just a little bit. I'll make a deal with you. If you open your mind about letting yourself remember a little, I'll open my mind so a husband can soon come into my life."

Her blue eyes relaxed. "Okay," she said.

Most people think a philosophical or psychological conversation is not possible with an Alzheimer's patient. I find it is possible. I heard from the social director that Selma was calmer after I left that day; there was some lasting effect.

A few months later, Selma passed away. She was beyond grief, fear, and pain. I was glad for our times together; I thought we had made some progress.

CHAPTER 6

Viola and Lolly

The following October 2001, I found two new sites as an adult school teacher at Holiday Manor and Sunrise. Here are two particular patients and how we were able to find our way to each other:

Viola is a woman I met at one of my first times at Holiday Manor. This facility is thirty years old and has about fifty residents. It seemed like a typical nursing home until I met the staff and the patients. I learned quickly that the residents here had hearts of gold. This Alzheimer's group, in the next two and a half years, became one of my most special group experiences.

At first, Viola didn't speak at all. She did open her arms in a gesture to hug me at the end of my session the first day, and she smiled a huge smile. I hugged her, looked into her eyes, took her hand and said, "Thank you for your acknowledgment and the recognition that you appreciate my being here." She gestured with her cheek to rub mine, cheek to cheek. I got her message.

The next week, Viola hummed, "La, la la la la." I looked at her and hummed "La La" back. That was our communication. One woman, Irvela, said to me, "I came to hear you, not to hear her singing." I said, "Those are her words for now to talk to me. I wanted to make sure she knew I heard her. It's a way to connect." Irvela understood.

When I had been at other sites, the Horizons and the Marriott, I found the residents just loved some of the old film performers. These memories involve their minds in positive recall. Whether they are recalling seeing these films forty or fifty years ago or if they are just being entertained by something familiar, it has a restorative effect on them in the present moment. One week, I showed some movies of Eddie Cantor and George Burns. At the end of the session, I asked the group, "Did anyone ever meet Eddie Cantor?" One woman answered from the audience, "I did. In Los Angeles I went to hear him sing."

Then from the other side of the room Viola spoke, "I did, too. In New York."

I was amazed Viola was speaking. "In New York?" I asked.

"Yes, Central Park."

"You went to hear him sing?"

She shook her head "no." I guessed. "He was there to hear you sing?"

She nodded. Then she looked up at me with a big smile, and said, "Good news."

"He brought you good news." I could only guess what the good news was. I asked, "Did he help you get your songs recorded?"

"Yes," she answered.

I didn't get the details but I assumed a contact was made. Then Viola broke into song. "On Blueberry Hill." I motioned for the group to chime in, and they did. "I found my thrill on Blueberry hill, la, la, la la."

For me, it was a victory. From no words, only gestures, to song, to dialogue. I had made a contact. I challenged myself each week to reach another person. Little by little, each week someone new opened up and shared his or her thoughts.

I feel lucky because my grandma and Uncle Bob helped me see that connection can be independent of words. I hope to bring to others a way to keep the connection alive through expressions, touch, song, memories, love.

Yes, there is a loss. But what is left can still be accessed. We can begin to see loved ones for what is still present in them.

Sunrise is a franchise of residential living. I was offering classes through the adult school in memory enhancement two times a week there to the Alzheimer's group and the regular residents. When Lolly arrived at Sunrise, she was very reticent; her daughter had just had lunch with her. Because Lolly was new to the home, and even though the Reminiscence Room is like a cozy living room, everything seemed strange, unfamiliar, without the warmth of her daughter's face and hand.

One week went by. I was informed that her medication had been changed; she was more relaxed—a little steadier and a little more talkative. By the third week, her personality was in full swing. She was playful, laughing. She and Oscar, another resident, were like little kids, playing and hitting each other with their elbows. She had completely transformed herself. She would make a grand entrance, as if she were showing off a new dress at the debutante ball when she was just entering the Reminiscence Room. I was thrilled to see her so happy. But then the activity director told me that now when her daughter came to visit, Lolly got tense, shutdown, and was tearful again. Now the problem with adjustment was the family members.

Instead of her family being as thrilled as I was that Lolly was safe, happy, and getting on well with her new resident friends, her family was resentful. I imagine this was because they felt jealous as much as they were pleased that "strangers" were helping her feel comfortable.

Cher, the activity director, loved and oversaw her residents like a mother hen, and really wanted to help the whole family heal together.

The important things are the safety, care, and well-being of the loved one. To stimulate the brain gives a new beginning and a new foundation to work from. If someone was a marathon runner and broke his or her leg, that runner wouldn't be expected to immediately run a marathon. And to focus on the loss doesn't help one in the recovery, doesn't offer his or her the motivation to develop strength again, go to physical therapy, eat the right foods, get the right exercises to build up and gain momentum. Perhaps a marathon may or may not be an option later, but look at all the other things that are possible: walking, swimming, and keeping company with loved ones. Those things help promote growth and healing.

An Alzheimer's person is the same. Focus on what is still present and work with that. In working with this group over the year we were together, I found them very alert and convivial. Later, we joined both the Alzheimer's group with the regular seniors. Everyone participated remarkably well. New people would come, some people died, but there was always a positive energy whenever I entered the place.

CHAPTER 7

All View

It was my first day as an adult memory enhancement instructor at a new facility, All View in Hollywood. The owner told me All View really stands for God. I was hugged and kissed by Shake, the social director. Shake said, "Thank you so much for coming. My heart is lifted." Shake put her hands over her heart. I had finally found a place where I fit. My ideas were welcomed, and I was embraced. Shake was an ex-flower child from the days in New York of Woodstock and Studio 54. She had a wonderful, nurturing and intuitive quality about her. She looked twenty years younger than she was, standing a slender five-foot six with short, reddish hair.

The Alzheimer's residents, my students, were huddled into the dining room. There were five square tables made of a walnut wood with matching chairs. More than half of the people were in wheelchairs. Even those who were ambulatory were sitting. I had a white board with new colored magic markers. I had written the word "Brainsprouts" on the board. Five of the staff members were present, which I liked because they'd be learning the memory system, too. As I looked out among the group, part of me panicked a little because after observing Shake's interactions with the residents, I realized that half of these people were nonverbal.

"Oh, my," I thought, "how will I be able to do this for two hours without feedback, at least the normal feedback, I had been used to?" I said to the group, "I want to explain a new concept to you: Brainsprouts." I took a deep breath, and the words came. "When we are first beginning to form in our mother's womb, our cells divide and develop our brain and our spinal cord. In our first year of life, neurons begin to make connections in our patterns of learning. We have billions and billions of neurons which form neural branches. They lay the foundation of our brain throughout our lives. The old medical model believed that whatever neurons we formed in our first six years of development stayed with us into old age. It was the belief that the brain was limited and couldn't grow further. So as we aged and lost brain cells, it would be natural for us to have memory loss. That was once considered a normal part of aging. How many of you believe in that old medical model?" (About half the people in the room raised their hands).

"It made sense, given that this is what our doctors and scientists told us. But years ago, I questioned that theory because on a daily basis, we grow skin cells, fingernails and toenails. Our hair grows. If we cut ourselves, within a few days the cut is healed. We get sick with colds, flu, other illnesses, and we get better. I kept wondering, "Why would the most powerful organ in our body not have the same regenerative capabilities as other parts of our body?" Now, all these years later, our doctors are saying they were misinformed, and we were misguided. The brain can regenerate from existing live cells. It is not just a natural part of aging to lose our memories. It's just not true. Now that we have this information, let's change our thinking to the new medical model: *our brains can regenerate.* We can continue to grow and learn throughout our entire lives. How many of you are willing to go with our new belief that the brain can grow?" Almost all of the responsive participants raised their hands. "Great," I said.

"Let's talk about something else. What is the most important thing we need to live besides oxygen, water, food, and exercise on the physical level? What is most important psychologically? What about our will? When I watched a yoga tape, 'The Power of Hatha Yoga,' the instructor, Nadder Shagagi, said that our will is more important than thought, because we will ourselves to think."

I gave an example of prisoners in a concentration camp. Many of the prisoners survived who had a passionate will to accomplish a goal after the war.

One woman said she wanted to come to America and raise a son to be an attorney. She did, and her son is a practicing attorney in Tarzana. Another lady said she lived to taste chocolate again or to see a beautiful sunset. Victor Frankl spoke of those prisoners in the camps who lost their will to live when the war that they'd hoped would be over by Christmas didn't end. Prisoners in the concentration camp during World War II would save their cigarettes to trade for bread or soup. However, when hope was lost, those prisoners reluctantly smoked their last cigarettes and were dead the next day.

They had given up their will and no longer believed they could continue to suffer without the end of the war in sight. According to Victor Frankl, it was having something purposeful to look forward to that gave individuals hope. Even Victor Frankl himself was able to maintain a bright spot of hope within himself, as did other prisoners even in the darkest of hours, if they had a vision. In fact, it is written in the Russian Bible, "Where there is no vision, the people perish."

I went around the room and asked each participant what he or she looked forward to. Felix, a slight man with white hair and a sweet smile, struggled a bit with his words, but finally, he was able to say, "My next hot meal." Millie, whose eyes had been closed up until that moment opened her eyes to say, "Dancing," and then she closed her eyes again. One man named Gus, who didn't have his teeth, wiggled his foot as he tried eagerly to form words. His utterances weren't quite distinguishable, but his eyes spoke to me as if to say, "Loved ones." He yearned for the company of those he had been closest to. Margaret, an alert, graying, tall woman still in good shape said, "Playing with Becker, the resident bloodhound."

I shared with the group my eagerness to be with them as something I looked forward to. "After all," I shared, "being in front of an audience with a microphone is one of my favorite things to do." They laughed. "All of us in this room have had full and active lives. When we are active and busy, it's easy to see our value. Now that that our lives are not as active as before, how do you see yourselves as valuable now?"

A few felt they didn't see their value. Others said they were valuable to their children. One woman said, "I am valuable to anyone who comes in contact with me." Another participant said, "I am of value to myself."

Jean spoke. She had a full head of white hair. She often had it styled, and she had makeup on her eyelids to set off her lovely blue eyes. I find her an amazing woman with grace and carriage at the age of ninety-three. "I was born in a covered wagon," she said. "I was the first born of seven brothers and sisters. I wrote a book called, *From the Covered Wagon to the Moon.*"

"I like that title, Jean," I said. "I'd love it if you'd bring the book in, and we can read it together." She said she didn't know where it was, but she'd ask her children.

"Imagine all that has happened since the covered wagon days," I suggested.

Margaret said, "We used to wash our clothes on a washboard and then hang them outside to dry."

"What state were you from?" I inquired.

"Minnesota," she said.

"How could you dry things in a cold winter? Wouldn't wet clothes turn into icicles?" She laughed. "No, the wind blew them dry."

Jean said, "It was too cold there. We didn't do much washing all winter. We'd wait 'til the spring. It was a struggle in those days. I ate trout because our wagon was set near a river. I didn't know there was any other kind of meat except trout for a long, long time. We had a grandma. Babe, we called her. She made great bread. It was delicious, and everyone would fight for a piece. I watched how she made it. Then, I started making it too. It was one of my first major accomplishments, besides having to look after my other brothers and sisters." Jean shared how much she liked school, told us stories of stagecoaches and gypsies. I like how she taught us.

Philip, who was new at the time and quite prolific, added an image we put on the board: a heart melting into another heart. He said that is what love is.

The next time I visited, Philip came to me. He was a slight man of about eighty; he had been in good spirits most of the time. He was talkative and often insightful. But this day, his shoulders were slumped. He said, "I am very depressed. My doctor just diagnosed me. I have Alzheimer's disease. I am sorry I missed your class."

"I understand, Philip. It was such a blow for you to take in the news that you didn't want to live. You needed to go to sleep."

"Yes, that's just how I feel. What can I do, especially at my age? I am only eighty-four and the worst thing of all …"

I finished his sentence. "The doctor said there is nothing he can do."

"Yes, that's exactly what he said. So what can you do when even the MDs from UCLA say there's nothing to do? I don't want to even face this. It's too terrible to think of."

"Philip, I don't want to take anything away from this shock you are presently experiencing. However, the class we had today, which was taped, is all about what you can do to help give energy and increase the speed and communication of the neurons that you still have left in your brain. We talked about neural branching."

"But what credentials do you have?" Philip asked. "You are not a doctor. How can you know something if the MD doesn't know?"

"It's my profession," I told him. "I've researched and studied over twenty years as a memory trainer in both education and corporations. I have a master's degree in psychology. I began my Alzheimer's work in 1985."

"Then, why don't they know?" He was really struggling.

"Philip, would you go to a bodybuilder if you wanted to learn exercises for your body or would you go to an MD?" I asked.

"Hmmm. Okay, talk to my family, please," Philip pleaded.

I set Philip up with one of the nurses to make sure he watched the video I showed in class so that he wouldn't have to wait two more days until I returned. I didn't want him to be anxious if it could be prevented.

Education helps reduce anxiety.

CHAPTER 8

Philip

The next day, February 13, I looked around the room at the participants from the All View site. The room is rectangular, adjacent to the kitchen and serves as a dining room. When one first enters All View on the ground floor, there is the sound of water from a feng-shui fountain, a lovely "bark hello" greeting from Becker and a new addition—a white, toy poodle. The office is just to the left of the entry way; then, down the hallway are the residents' rooms in the decor of old Hollywood. The rooms even have Hollywood names. The facility is two stories high and has about thirty residents.

This day, there was a new man named Art. He was slightly balding, about five-foot six, slender except for a little potbelly. His face had angular features and nice cheekbones. But all I could feel looking at him was his distress. Art was anxious, disoriented, and crying. He did not remember why he was in the assisted living center. He cried, "What did I do? What did I do to deserve this?" It is very important as a family to discuss with the Alzheimer's loved one your concerns about their needs—that you want them safe and attended to, and that you love them. Ask them how they'd feel about being with other people during the day while you are at work. Tell them of your concerns about them getting lost if they go out, or if they forget to turn off the stove, or if something happened you wouldn't be there right away to help. Let your loved one share his or her feelings.

See ways that you can get him or her support while you work in the form of a caregiver during the day or a day care center with activities. Try that if you can. If it comes to the point that you feel assisted living is the way to go, then see if you can go first for lunch and meet and greet others. See if your loved one can go for the day for a fee and see how he or she feels.

Reassure your loved one that you are most concerned for their safety and well-being and that you feel you want to provide the best care for them and that you will be there often to visit and take them out to be with you and family. In some places, you can still spend the night together. I think these are good ways to transition.

Be honest and truthful about your needs, his or her needs, your care and concerns. Make sure their room away is filled with family pictures, familiar items, just like when you have a son or daughter go away to camp or to college. Let your loved one know that you want to try it out and see if it's a working alternative to being alone at home or without supervision that is needed now that the illness is present or has progressed.

If you don't communicate, your loved one may feel lost, scared, confused, abandoned. He or she may question what did they do wrong? Why are they being punished to be "put away" from their home and family? This is a tragic feeling. Even though the memory is impaired, the loved one still has all the same needs for love, connection, contact, socialization, communication, touch, and support. Isolation is one of the biggest complaints that doctors speak about when they talk of their patients in nursing homes or in assisted living homes.

It is scary enough to have a diagnosis of having a memory problem. That alone can create more anxiety, insecurity, and fear. That is the time to ensure that the truth is discussed and the trust of the family is ever present. This way he or she can be secure they are not being left or abandoned. The decision to be placed in an alternative home is for their best care, and you want them to feel assured, reassured, safe, and comfortable. Let them know when you are coming. Write it down so they can see it on a calendar. Help them use the memory pictures to imagine your visits, the touch, the sound, the feelings, and the picture of it. If you are going to go on an outing, help them picture the location and the activities in their mind, (Just like the chapter where I spoke about Bert remembering when his wife is coming to pick him up.) This will give your loved one the anticipation of your visit, just like when one is looking forward to a date, a party, a trip, a dinner, something important to you.

The key is to make sure your loved one stays close, connected, and aware that he or she is still wanted and loved by you. Personally, I feel truth is the best way to handle this situation. Others feel if they tell the truth, they won't get the cooperation they are looking for. Yet, the distress a loved one feels when abandoned in a strange place is pure torture. To feel safe in any situation, I find truth works the best.

I discussed this with Cher, a social director of another assisted living center, Rising Moon. She said that she always encourages the families to be honest. False truths, false hopes cause more confusion in an already confused mind. It's just too difficult for the loved one to think, and this creates more havoc in their brains, in their emotions. The few reserves they have are depleted by trying to figure out, "Why the hell did my family dump me with a bunch of strangers?"

Philip, on the other hand, knew where he was and wanted to do something to help himself. Earlier, Philip had asked me to contact his daughter in Boston. I did so. He had told me that he recognized he might need an additional source of nutrition since he'd been depressed and hadn't been eating well. I knew a doctor who is both an MD and a nutritionist whom I trust. Before I could even discuss this with Philip's daughter, she blocked any means of support I had to offer. She screamed, "I am not taking him to any more doctors! He slips and slides like this all the time. He knows he has dementia. It isn't anything new. Maybe he just forgot. He takes nosedives like this all the time. He's just been on a honeymoon at All View these last two months." She continued to express her frustration and ended her conversation with, "It's nice you care about my dad and want to give him time. I'm frustrated. I just don't know what to do, but thanks anyway."

Never once did she offer to take my support. I was dismayed. She doesn't know what to do, yet won't take what I can offer. I realized the patient isn't just in the hands of caring practitioners. He or she can be in the hands of the family who may yearn and wish for, but don't always do the best for their loved one. Philip hadn't been at class the last two sessions. I wondered if he'd plummeted again. Did he have anything to look forward to which is enough for him to want to get up again?

"Where is Philip?" I asked Dawn, a caregiver. "He's in his bed. He's in Room 208."

"In here," Philip called from inside his room. I saw Philip lying on his little single bed across the room near a window. He was curled up.

"I've gone downhill," he said.

"Yes, I know you took a nosedive," I responded.

"That's exactly it, a nosedive." He winced. "Ever since I talked to the doctor, I've been down."

"Yes, you gave up, Philip," I confirmed.

"You're right. I have given up. What is it that I'm fighting for now? It's a losing battle."

"I don't think your doctor gave you all the facts." I wanted him to hear me clearly. Philip looked at me intently. He walked with a cane a few weeks ago, but this week, he was resigned to a walker. He was slightly balding in the front, but he had most of the rest of his hair. He spoke clearly in full sentences without hesitation. He didn't seem at all like someone with Alzheimer's. Maybe he had some form of dementia, but in this conversation it wasn't apparent.

"Philip, I taped a KCET special on the newest information about the brain. I brought it so you can hear ALL THE FACTS about the brain. Then, you can make your own decision. Right now, you've rolled over, based on half the facts. I want you to see the whole picture." I could tell he was listening. "The whole class is waiting for you, Philip, so we can watch this together."

Philip's body said "yes" even before his mouth said "okay." He was already sitting up on his bed when he asked me to position his walker for him. As we walked down the hallway, he said to me, "I've been thinking. I need a supercharged vitamin." I had talked to him a week before about nutritional supplements; I had told him to check with his doctor. I'm glad the suggestion took hold.

Once we got to the room where we hold class, Philip sat with the others and watched. The first part of the film showed a doctor saying how doctors were wrong about their theories of the brain, up until now. *The brain can continue to grow and regenerate into our adult and senior years.* I echoed, "*Wrong … See the doctors were wrong.* They admitted it themselves." I addressed the group, but I especially wanted Philip to hear it too.

The next powerful image in the film was an experiment. A substance was administered to mice, which wiped out neurons from parts of their cerebral cortex. The experimenters were amazed to see under a microscope that stem cells came in and filled the area that had been destroyed. Also, they came in the exact location where they were needed, and then dendrites grew to make neural connections in the entire region. The data concluded that the brain could regenerate completely. This amazed the scientists, because before this there had never been medical proof of these brain phenomena. Some of the other participants in the group were also happy to be made aware of this new information about the brain. It's one thing when I tell them and draw little pictures on the board of the brain regeneration. But it's quite different for them to be hearing it directly from medical doctors from Einstein College, UC Irvine, the Salk Institute, and other noted universities. It substantiates what I have been discussing with them.

Art began crying again. He asked if I could drive him home. At this point, I had a group of about ten people in the room. Some of the wanderers had left after the video completed. I thought I'd use this as an opportunity to see if the group could offer any support to Art, because each person in the room had given up his or her home and lifestyle when he or she moved here. Unfortunately, the nonverbal people couldn't offer much verbal support but could definitely feel compassion. I saw this in their eyes. Louise, not a resident, who sees her husband twice a week, spoke up. She had tears in her eyes. "I miss my husband. I am all alone in the house now."

This is the other side of the loss. "I come to visit at least twice a week just to be with him. But the emotions of leaving and the days in between are tremendously difficult. We've been married fifty-eight years. I don't understand." Louise said. "My husband was a vegetarian, took mounds of vitamins, even had Chelation treatments. It makes no sense to either one of us that he would get Alzheimer's disease." I was curious, too. I asked if he had ever had a hair analysis.

She said, "No." I would be curious even now what those results would be, if there is any metal toxicity or nutritional deficiency that would show up. Later, Louise shared with me that Felix had suffered a heart attack years before. It was after the heart attack he changed his diet. Prior to that he ate "all the wrong foods," she shared.

I could see this was a compatible couple. They were always happy to be in each other's company. I saw the love in their eyes. Yet, Felix, her husband, as sweet as he is, clearly has lost most of his abilities except for a few words and loving gestures of touch and rubbing with his hands.

I think of companionship. Art's new loss of home and the life he had known. Philip's decision whether to fight for his life, and if so, what makes it worth fighting for? His wife had died, but he had a girlfriend, Rose, whom the director of All View brought for a visit. Philip's daughter was going to be visiting from Boston for a few days with his grandson. He seemed a little bit apprehensive because he didn't want his grandson to see him depleted, but he also seemed pleased to know he was going to get the attention of the visit. He would have liked his sons to call and visit more often. Of course, he wanted his super-boost vitamin too. Philip did seem better after the video. The color returned to his cheeks, and his spirit seemed a bit better. Knowledge is a powerful tool.

The following Monday at All View, I noticed Philip wasn't in class. When I finished the program that day, I walked into his room. "Hi, Philip I heard that you had visitors this week. I heard your daughter came. How was it?"

"Did my daughter come? I don't remember." I asked him some questions, but he said, "I don't need an interrogation, I didn't invite you in here. Please leave." I was astonished and really hurt; I walked out to ask the social director what happened. He told me Philip's doctor told him that his cancer was spreading. It had gone into his liver. He truly wasn't feeling well.

I felt a stomachache the next few hours and thought maybe this is a type of distress Philip was in. Perhaps I was having sympathy pains. I saw a card in a shop. It was a picture by Van Gogh of a man laying his head in his hands. I bought it, thinking I'd give it to Philip. I'd say in the card, "This man is feeling it for you, Philip, so you don't have to feel such anguish."

When I got home, I thought about it and realized that perhaps Philip wouldn't get the communication because the staff would misinterpret my actions. I decided to just walk in with a smile the next week and visit him.

(Next week)

I did and I knocked his door. "Help me. Please help me," he pleaded.

"What can I do, Philip?" I asked.

"Who is that?" he inquired.

"It's Vicki." I called out.

"Oh, Vicki, could you please get me some water?"

Philip was lying on the bed on his side. He just had on a pair of boxer shorts. His face was swollen, as were his hands. I could see he couldn't even sit up. I reassured him. I would get him some water. I did.

I sat on the bed and leaned over to him so that I could securely grip the glass while he sipped. I bent the straw closer to his mouth. "I feel such heartburn," he anguished.

"What is it that I have? What is it the doctor said?"

As a "teacher," I am not allowed to divulge information.

"Here." I was just giving him water. "Please," he asked, "give me something to help the heartburn." I left him and went to see the manager who said, "He's always dying lately." Then I went to the nurse, who said she'd give him his medication and then see how he felt. Why couldn't she just get an antacid for him and take it up now? Why must he wait in agony? I was running late. I left, not going back up to say good-bye to Philip. I was too frustrated to have to hear his pleas to run back empty-handed, with only assurances someone would be up soon.

Monday morning, I walked in. "Philip passed away this weekend." It was just three days since I had seen him. I was relieved that he was out of pain. They had brought hospice in on Friday and set him up on morphine. He had his birthday on March 14. He turned eighty-three. He died on Saturday, March 16. His girlfriend, Rose, had come to see him, as had his family.

The manager said, "It's interesting everyone came to see him when he had his birthday. Then, he was gone." The social director said, "Yes, it was fast. The minute the doctor told him that he was going to die, that his cancer had spread, he went downhill fast.

I wondered to myself if Philip had given up first and then the cancer spread like wildfire, or did the cancer spread first? I wonder if his mind willed himself to die, because as he said, "What is there left to fight for?"

CHAPTER 9

You Stir My Soul

It was a Tuesday. Although the sky was only a little gray, my internal sun wasn't shining. I was still struggling with my own brain injury and my own loneliness, wanting to finish graduate school, recover my brain. It was hard for me sometimes with the difficulties I was going through. Fortunately it helped to have a therapist to listen to me and provide support. Not having any family and my brother being so far away, I am fortunate to have my wonderful Siamese kitty, Sasha, who has been my friend and companion since she was two months old. I walk her on a leash, and we have traveled together. So I didn't feel so alone during emotionally difficult times.

As I walked into Holiday Manor, the first person I saw was Richard. He is a small man and seems young to me. All his brown hair frames a rather rugged face. His sometimes-smile was nowhere to be seen. "Tough day to be alive," I said to him.

He shot me in make-believe, turning his fingers into a pretend-gun.

"Easier to be dead today than to feel anything," I said. He nodded his head and smiled. I knew how he felt. It wasn't hard. I was feeling the same way.

I looked around the room. Marian, who has white hair and lovely blue eyes, sat slumped in her wheelchair. I imagined it must be difficult to sit so many hours propped up like that without exercising or even stretching out all her limbs in a nice swimming pool.

Margaret, whose face often tells me the emotional tone of the room through her smile, her rapt attention, or her head down, dozing off, had a flat face today, her eyes looking nowhere.

Bernice, whose eyes let me know right away whether her daughter had been visiting over the weekend by either a glow that lights up her whole face or just a monotone look, stared straight ahead.

"It's a tough day, I think, for everyone." Their eyes looked up at me, telling me I read the room correctly. "Some days are better, and some days are more difficult. This is one of those more difficult days. I imagine it must feel crummy to be in a wheelchair today. I sense it's a sad feeling not to be able to just get up and run or jog. It's been years since you've been able to act on passionate feelings, making love or just going out for a walk around the block."

Their eyes looked at me like, "How did you know?"

"You know, when I was little, I thought God had feelings the way I did. I had an older brother who needed lots of attention. I had the chicken pox when I was five years old. We lived in Tucson, Arizona, and he was having difficulty with his third grade studies. My mom and dad got him a tutor. They were busy with him, and I sensed it, so if I needed something I was shy about asking, because I thought they were already tired from his demands.

"After a while, I'd feel lonely and left out so I'd cry. My mom thought I was just tired. She'd say I needed a nap. Or she thought I needed to eat. She didn't recognize it was my emotional frustration that I wanted to feel attended to and important just like my brother. So, when it rained, I thought that God was feeling frustrated too, just like me, and he had to shed his tears of frustration."

Margaret smiled, she beamed. "How cute to think God thought like you." Renee said, "That's how a five year-old would think." Maybe she didn't even say it but said it with her eyes and her nod. We were all on the same wavelength. I continued, "In fact, I thought that whatever weather we were having, God was expressing his feelings. When it was sunny, he was happy, windy— moody and playful, torrents of rain— raging and argumentative, cloudy—getting ready to either cry, feel sad, frustrated, or disappointed. Therefore, God set the precedent that it's okay for us to feel all of our feelings.

"Yet, in our society we can only be happy or sick, right? Most people don't want to know about emotions like, sadness, loneliness, distress, and misery. They like us if we are happy and loving, but say to us when we're sad, 'Well, I hope you feel better soon,' then we'll get together. It's like sending the message that we are not okay and can't be with others if we aren't feeling positive emotions."

"That's right," Irvela chimed in.

"But it's not fair, is it? We need to be held and paid attention to and comforted even more in times of distress. Those are hard emotions to hold alone," I said.

"That's why we all come together here. We join one another and through our community, our family here, we can all get along." Helen from Boston spoke.

I smiled and said, "Yes. We have each other. And you help me too. When I come to you, I feel received and accepted. That gives me comfort."

"I'm glad," Barbara and Bernice said. Irvela seconded it. Helen bowed and smiled.

"We've talked a lot over the last few weeks about difficult emotions. We've discussed Earnest Hemingway and his emotions of both great love and great torment when he loved another woman besides his wife. We watched Van Gogh anguish over getting an accurate portrayal of the sun in his paintings, as if it were melting the canvas the way it melted the sky that day. He'd cry over his work not being sold, yet relished the brilliance of red. It's all our emotions that give life to creative work, whether it is writing or painting."

Helen said, "I am just a little worm. It would be too difficult to be a genius. Yet, I can appreciate what they've given us."

"When we see a painting of a pretty picture it makes us feel nice and warm. Yet, when we see a painting of a raging storm, with a faint sun reemerging, it gives us something to grab—to think about. It gives us room to have the emotions if someone is showing us his or hers."

"You stir my soul," Irvela said.

"It's necessary for us to embrace each other and ourselves through all the range of our emotions. Even terror," I stated. "What do we do when we have terror? We get too scared to move to do anything. We curl up in a little ball and hold tight. When we have a young child with us, we reassure that child and extend a hand and then he or she is safe. We are here. But how do we reassure ourselves as terrified adults?"

We had never gone this far emotionally. We'd never gone to the place where all of us in the room stopped. I looked out. Still the group was with me. We were still together.

I concluded, "All we can do is try anything to make ourselves feel safe. I bet that's what happened to all of you in here at one time or another. You just couldn't cope anymore with the losses of loved ones, spouses; you got scared, terrified and put yourselves here to be safe."

All the heads nodded. I had hit it. I've known this! Deep in each Alzheimer's person was a stopping place, because he or she couldn't feel safe enough to move forward without a support system to give them the safety they'd had before.

"It's true for us all," I assured them.

"Yet, within this time of our sharing safely, our loving connection, and space to feel our feelings, we may be able to step forward into an unknown together."

Margaret said, "Yes," in a very soft voice. I bent down to hear her saying. "And this time it will be different."

CHAPTER 10

Insight into the Illness

The idea of a life becoming so changed with a loss of support that the fear causes a person to actually stop their life and unconsciously or consciously lose hope was first revealed to me when I contemplated what happened to my grandmother in the last fifteen years of her life.

Our Grandma Ida had been living with us in Tulsa for about six months because Grandpa Harry died on Memorial Day in 1963. Gary and I had lost our grandfather; my mother lost her dad; Grandma, her husband. For my dad, Grandpa was the best babysitter he could ever find. My dad told me years later, that he looked out the window one afternoon, watching Grandpa playing with my brother and me, giving us rides in the wheelbarrow. He was amazed how deeply Grandpa loved us. Perhaps even more than my own father was capable of.

My mom was a great cook and big on the family having dinner together, although on some days, she'd let my brother and me have dinner in front of the television to watch cartoons. It had been a trying day for Mom with her two children: Gary, my brother, who was twelve at the time, and I, her Poojoo (my mother's pet name for me), was nine. We'd all sat down for a Thursday dinner

They Can Still Remember To Love

at home. It was a wonderful brisket with green beans, which had been one of Grandpa's favorites. Daddy liked it too. Mom served us as we were seated at the round, pink kitchen table. About five minutes into the meal, Grandma burst into tears. "Tucktah."

"Tucktah" means "my love" in Yiddish. Mother scolded her. "It's been six months. You didn't even get along that well. You were often arguing. It's enough already." I couldn't believe my ears. My mother never spoke that way.

I don't blame my mom for her frustration. It was her loss too. Grandma was having too hard a time at the table to eat and left for her room. I don't remember if I finished my meal or excused myself, but I was concerned about Grandma.

I walked down the one step into her room. She was sitting quietly and teary-eyed, looking at a picture of Grandpa. Her feet were dangling over the edge of the bed like a young girl; only she was about sixty-five at the time. Her green eyes were red from crying, imagining a life without him.

Grandma had met Grandpa when she was seventeen. They had both immigrated to America from Poland, never to see their parents again. I was remembering the story she told me of their first kiss. It had begun to rain. She and Grandpa were walking. "He was so handsome." He ushered her under an awning, opened the umbrella, and once both of them were under it, he bent down and gave her a kiss. "Our first kiss." She smiled as she told me; she brightened, as if remembering the scene brought him back, alive, even for a moment.

I sat down next to Grandma on the bed.

"It's okay," I tried to reassure her, "to cry that Grandpa's gone."

Grandma looked at me and said, "Mawmy said no." (That was how she pronounced mommy, "Maw–mee" with her Polish accent).

I said, "Mommy's wrong!" It was very risky to defy my mother. It could mean she'd take away her special love for me. My mother could control me with a look. If she gave me "the look," I was already crushed, but in this moment I was outside of time. Something important was happening that night between

Grandma and me. We had a magical relationship; I felt I was the one that could speak to her. Who else would? I spoke affirmatively; no one else could hear us.

I looked at her. I was so young I didn't know all that she was feeling. I couldn't put together what it felt like for her missing his warmth at night, his touch, his voice, and his face. I just knew the backyard wasn't the same without Grandpa pushing me on the rope swing or watching me dive into the water in the little swimming pool he built for me.

"Grandma, cry, it's okay, I miss Grandpa too."

In retrospect, I realized something changed that night. Grandma, who had been very expressive and emotional, began suppressing her feelings. Whether it was conscious or not, Grandma shut down. I think she did it to be a lighter burden for my mother. My mom couldn't afford to feel her own pain. She had two kids to raise, a household to run, as well as caring for her mother. Although she tried to hide it, my mom wasn't well.

She'd had a thyroidectomy when she was twenty-two. The doctors took out too much of her thyroid gland. She suffered from mexidema, migraines, and fatigue. It caused my mother anxiety to see her mother distressed. But I was Grandma's only granddaughter, and she adored me. One time when I was five, Grandma said to me, as she was going into the shower to put some color rinse onto her red hair, "Would you like a little touch of red in your hair like grandma's?" I thought that sounded fun. So, I got in the shower with her, and she shampooed in some red dye. We laughed. Later, my mother scolded Grandma. Grandma said, "Let her be a little redhead like me. It just washes out." I liked it. But Mommy didn't.

Memories of Grandma: walking outside in the backyard to kick a ball and sing to the birds. She sewed my ice-skating outfits. One time, I made a clay vase at school. I thought it was weird-looking, and my mom said, "Grandma would love it!" My mom sent it to her. Three months later, I received a first prize ribbon in the mail. Grandma had entered my vase in a Pacific Ocean Park contest. I won first place. I was thrilled. She could see my creativity.

I didn't. She loved me and always greeted me with a smile and a warm hug for her "angel face."

Here's a poem she wrote me for my third birthday:

To Vicki on Her Birthday

> Today you are three years old;
> The glitter of diamonds,
> The shimmer of gold
> Can't compare with the smile
> That you unfold.
> I wish I could hold you
> And whisper in your ear,
> "I love you, Angel Face,
> I love you, dear."
> I'd like to dance with you
> And whirl you around as before,
> And hear you say, as you often did,
> "Grandma, dance some more."
> And when we'd stop to get some rest,
> I would hug you to my breast;
> To do again these little things,
> I'd fly to you like a bird on wings.
> MANY, MANY HAPPY BIRTHDAYS, VICKI, DEAR

Grandma Berg Adele Ida, 1957

Grandma moved out later in 1964 to go to Los Angeles. She still visited us, and we went to Los Angeles to visit her, but it was never the same without Grandpa.

Eight years later, when I was seventeen and my brother was twenty, he and I drove to Los Angeles from Denver. My mother, newly divorced, moved to Denver to be closer to me. Our mom was very generous; she gave us her Chrysler, money, and AAA tour book. She wanted my brother and me to have time together, since he'd already had a year away at college. She wanted us to stay close.

Gary and I had a lovely time traveling to the Grand Canyon, Las Vegas, through the great parks of Yosemite and Sequoia. Then, we made it to our final destination, Los Angeles, and stayed with Grandma.

Staying with her this time was odd. We noticed the *Yellow Pages* in the freezer, candles in the refrigerator. Much of the food in the refrigerator had rotted. Each night, Grandma would come into the kitchen in the middle of the night and pull out the refrigerator plug. She often forgot to put it back in the morning, hence the rotting food. She said she didn't like the noises the refrigerator made.

When my brother and I noticed these peculiarities, we asked her about them. It made perfect sense to her why *Yellow Pages* belonged in the freezer—to hold the food in place. The candles in the fridge would prevent melting. The refrigerator noises scared her at night, so of course, she'd pull the plug.

Grandma had always been a little paranoid. My mom said it was because of the trauma she survived as a child. Grandma had to leave her parents at the age of thirteen to come to America with her brother and sisters, never to see her parents again. One time when Grandma and my brother Gary and I were at a local deli having a meal, she was afraid the salt and pepper shakers were bugged. My mom said this was because of the fear of the Cossacks and the midnight beatings that used to happen in Poland. Gary and I thought without Grandpa's warmth to give her comfort, these fears were heightened.

This was around 1973. She entered a nursing home about three years later. Grandma loved nature. She loved to take walks and wander. She got kicked out of two nursing homes because of her appreciation of nature; she'd wander off to smell the flowers and watch the birds, spending hours walking on the grounds. The final nursing home kept her strapped into a wheelchair. Shortly after that, she lost all muscle tissue and her ability to walk. Then, she had a catheter put into her. It's easier for the nursing home staff that way. Nature was the last true joy for Grandma; her demise began when she was no longer able to enjoy nature.

I remember the last time I went to see her in 1979. She was in her wheelchair in the TV room area of Sun Slope Residential Living in San Fernando Valley. Grandma had a tissue in one hand and was trying to grab the back of the chair of the woman in front of her. She thought the woman was her sister, Sonia. She was saying in a very soft moan, "Sonia, Sonia."

"Hi, Grandma." I grinned, as I had always greeted her. She looked at me. Although she couldn't say my name, I recognized the love in her eyes; she knew I was someone who made her heart sing. I rolled her outside, catheter and all, sang her songs she used to sing to me as a child. I talked to her about the birds, reminded her of how she loved nature. In my backyard in Tulsa, she had shared with me about how beautiful God was, how lovely the birds, the trees, and the flowers were. We sang and clapped hands. For me, it was wonderful that the essence of her was still so much alive.

It was a good feeling to give back the love and appreciation she'd given me. I recited to her another poem she had written to me on my third birthday.

> *Lovely is my Vicki like the sun across the sea.*
> *Lovely is my Vicki I hope she thinks of me.*
> *Summer, winter, spring, and fall, God made the seasons.*
> *To love Vicki one doesn't need reasons.*
> *Lovely is my Vicki like the morning dew*
> *Lovely is my Vicki I wish to be with you.*
> *To have our moments and joy of little things*
> *I'd fly to you like a bird on wings.*

Grandma died a few months later. She didn't die of Alzheimer's but of pneumonia, which is what happens to many. The doctors didn't describe her illness as Alzheimer's but as "multiple sclerosis of the brain."

I thought back wondered when her decline began. It dawned on me. It was the night "Mawmy" said "no." There went the expressive grandma who had to stifle her grief over the loss of Grandpa and the life she had known.

Although her illness was physical, it had emotional components. In Grandma's case, I feel it was triggered by her deep loss, which wasn't fully grieved. The mind shuts down; the fear and pain become so great that one's thinking changes. Thus over time, physical deterioration begins. This is the first time I tracked the idea that emotions are a precursor which affect the brain so much that the body can become physically ill.

I believe that a much higher percentage of people than is recognized begin to lose brain function because of an emotional onset that triggers loss, depression from grief, or whatever kind of loss is suffered. Then, as the thinking changes, the brain chemistry changes; thus, the physical deterioration begins. The body becomes more prone to an invasion by foreign substances or bacteria because the immune system has weakened and cannot stay strong to fight off invaders.

Some forms of dementia also may develop because of nutritional issues. A person may not feel like eating which can lessen the nutritional balance of his or her diet. Living in a stable environment filled with regular meals, socialization, exercises, and activities allows regular rhythms for the body to adjust to a life-changing shift.

Our emotional needs, our need for a sense of purpose, for stimulation of body and mind, for a sense of self, even for sexual relationships and companionship may vary, but those are core needs and are vital to our joy and happiness no matter how the body ages.

CHAPTER 11

The Making of a Champion

When I was in graduate school at Antioch in the late 1990s, many new studies came out about depression causing memory loss. In fact, Dr. Andrew Leuchter, a noted psychiatrist at UCLA, changed his focus a few years ago from dementia to depression. If you can help the depression, then the deterioration can perhaps be lessened.

One of the difficulties I find in our culture is that individuals, as well as groups as a whole, don't know how to deal with death: talk about it, discuss it, or feel it. There cannot be a time line on grieving. It's individual. Each person handles it differently. One may grieve for twenty-eight years and someone else four months. It depends on what the individual needs. Yet many of us will respond to a loved one with, "Well, besides the death of your husband, mother, father, brother, sister, lover, relative, (you fill in the blank), how's the rest of your life going?" You may laugh reading this, but it's true. Aside from that, Mrs. Lincoln, how did you like the show?

However, there are wonderful grief support groups that one can stay in as long as needed to emote, feel, express, cry— whatever is needed to move forward.

Once one has moved forward, what is needed is a support system: Those individuals in one's life who say, "Yes, you're great."

We all need to feel acceptance, approval and a sense of importance. At least, I know I do, and that doesn't change at any age.

Dealing with grief is individual. Sometimes, grief isn't just one loss or two, but many. However, spending the time to process the grief and using the opportunity to share and heal it, may actually improve one's health rather than allowing the sadness or denial to cause possible memory or mental health problems later. Sometimes, waves crash and hit so hard that there is hardly time to come up for a breath before another wave crashes and takes you under. Here is a story of one of my own long-standing issues that continued for over a decade or more.

My brother and I are very close. When I wanted to move to NYC, I asked him if that was a good idea. He told me he loved me and I was his sister, and I was valuable to him. I would be even more valuable if I lived in New York. So I moved there in 1989 from San Diego. Gary and I talked a lot and decided we wanted to be closer to each other. He moved from Denver and joined me in NYC in 1991. He'd always handled the family trust. Whatever monies and properties had been in the family were lost, both due to the oil crash of the late 1980s and my brother's illness. Whatever decisions we'd had to make, we had no father or support to assist us. Within two weeks of his arrival at my home, he had a nervous breakdown. That's when his illness was fully diagnosed.

After eight months of living with my brother, my Epstein-Barr flared up. He moved out and ended up living in a basement apartment in Queens. I moved to Queens too to keep an eye on him.

I watched the television show *Quantum Leap* reruns starring Scott Bakula nightly when I was teaching as the only special education teacher at Monroe high school with difficult students at 186th Street in the Bronx. We had to leave school by 2:30 p.m. for our safety, to give you an idea of the neighborhood. Most of my students thought they would be dead or in jail by the time they were twenty-five. They thought learning was a waste of their time, and I should buy new boots because one of mine had a little hole in the front. I would go to bed at 10:00 p.m. and wake up to watch *Quantum Leap* at 11:00 p.m. That TV show was the only soothing part of my life. It was the only thing that made me feel good. After a year and a half at Monroe, I transferred to an alternative high school, but it wasn't much better. The students were rude and mean, just mean. I was assaulted by a female student. I decided to return to my dream of acting in film and television. I finally got out of New York to go to Los Angeles in 1996. My brother had stabilized. Then, I incurred injuries from being whipped around on a "Back to the Future" ride at Universal Studios in 1998.

There was also a terrible automobile crash: I was hit three times by a semi-truck in 1999. My car was totaled, but I lived. I was left brain-injured. Yes, the memory person was left without a memory. I had a job in Norwalk at the time, teaching English to ninth graders. After a few days, I tried to return to school, but the principal had already hired a substitute. I actually thought I could immediately resume teaching until I walked into the classroom to get some of my belongings and honestly couldn't remember who my students were and who weren't.

The doctors told me I'd never teach again. My neck and brain couldn't hold up against stress and tension from classroom management conflict, they said. I felt unaccustomed to myself. I had no ability to hold on to me. I was shaking all the time. It was frightening to drive. If I was on the freeway near a semi-truck, I became so frightened my body turned cold from my chest all the way down to my toes. I prayed to make it through, pass the truck, and continue on the highway until I could find my way safely home.

"Find" is really the word. I got lost a lot during those first three years. I even got lost on my way to the chiropractor I had been seeing for twenty-five years. I'd miss exits, forget turns. If it rained, I'd shake and do my best not to have to drive. I lost my ability to focus. When I'd try to answer a question in graduate school or even write a paper, I was speaking in circles.

On an evaluation, one professor suggested I should take a course in public speaking to learn to organize my thoughts. Eventually, that evaluation was disregarded when I met with the teacher privately and explained to her that I had been a professional public speaker for over twenty-five years, speaking both nationally and internationally. What she was witnessing was a brain-injured woman trying to continue getting her master's.

Fortunately, I had completed most of my course work and was able to manage my other courses through weekend workshops, then put a paper together. The papers were two pages. Over time, I could, with other people helping me to edit, handle that. Thank goodness my ten- to twelve-page research papers and theory papers had already been completed. I couldn't drop out of school and still graduate within the time frame I needed to match my disability support. I couldn't work and go to school again, not until I had healed from my injuries. I knew this would take time, years in fact—six years it took to come back to most of my self. It took four years to hold my neck up without a neck brace or chronic spasms from disc herniations and bulges.

The last thing a brain-injured person wants to deal with is memory. It's too hard. First, it was too hard to remember. The body is slow to process. Just to tolerate the difficulty of thinking from one step to another and one thought to another takes all one's energy. I could finally understand how my special education students had to process their thinking slowly; I needed to be patient. They could answer, but I had to wait, let their brains take the time needed to come up with the answer to a problem.

The second difficulty was to face a memory problem when I had a superlative memory. I wasn't who I was. I was sad to be in chronic physical and mental pain. I had to heal more first emotionally until I could deal with the woman I'd become. It was scary. I did know the right holistic practitioners who could eventually help me. I knew I could continue my research. I also knew I had to get better. I had future patients, a future as a therapist and as a memory therapist. I had a book to write and finish. What the doctors—the "regular" MDs—were telling me was that I was as good as I would get or I knew too much for my own good that I needed to just relax go on a date to a movie and take care of myself. But that wasn't good enough for me.

Through a combination of treatments by Dr. Timothy Binder (a living legend who trained in homeopathic and naturopathic treatments and studied acupuncture in China as well) including Chelation treatments, acupuncture, vitamin nutrition, yoga, exercises, psychotherapy, hair analysis, and working with my memory training methods with my patients, I moved forward.

In addition, Dr. Harold Toomin, a neuropathic scientific engineer in Los Angeles suggested I do biofeedback and get a SPECT scan, and he was able to retrace exactly what happened in the truck accident and to identify the injuries with accuracy. Through this, he helped me know I needed more oxygen and my own memory training methods which would be best for me to teach senior groups memory. That way, I'd be practicing and so would they. They were slow, and so was I. We would heal together. He made a treatment plan for me that was perfect. From July 2000 until February 2003, I worked with nine different Alzheimer's and senior facilities and assisted living centers, running memory training classes. Not only did I help the patients, I helped myself recover.

Needless to say after such a difficult decade, I felt tattered and worn. The Alzheimer's groups supported me emotionally as did my therapist, classmates, and a few longtime friends.

The summer of 2003, I went to my forty-year Camp Agawak reunion weekend in Minocqua, Wisconsin. There I remembered the "me" I had been most of my early life before losses, deaths, divorces, betrayals, and abandonments—all the issues of my twenties, thirties, and forties. My old camp friends recognized me immediately after thirty years. I was remembered as the beautiful girl with the big brown eyes. I felt sought after. I was remembered, truly remembered in a way I hadn't been aware of.

Other campers, now either grandmothers or mothers of twenty-year-olds, came to me. Kathy Burke, who was only a year younger than me, said, "I remember you as a goddess."

"A goddess?" My goodness, I was flattered. I had never considered myself that. Certainly, no man had treated me that way. She said, "I remember those beautiful doe eyes, brown, full like a little deer and so sweet, sensitive, and you were such a great athlete." I was touched.

In our first morning of the camp reunion, I went to the field. I ran straight to the archery range. I watched a few people shoot; and then, it was my turn. I remembered exactly how to put in the feathered arrow into the bow, how to aim, pull and let go. I hit the target! Then, I shot another arrow. Bull's-eye! I heard myself say to me, "You're great! You're great!" I proceeded to continue my practice, about five rounds in all—five bull's-eyes later, my self-esteem rose. I had me back.

I shared in conversation with Mona Hecht of my accident, losses and recovery. Mona looked at me and said, "Vicki, you are a champion!" A champion? I thought about it the whole night. The next day at breakfast I said, "Mona, thank you so much for saying I am a champion. I feel it."

"You are!" she said.

"I believe it. I do." A champ is one who is great, who excels, gets whipped, defeated, comes back, again and again, get whipped again and again, comes back and triumphs.

I was able to take all that had happened to me and call it "my development." Becoming a champion: I hold that inside me. That means there is no room in my life anymore for those who are negative.

Truly, when I think of my seniors, I see the spirit of champions in them too! Each one of them gives something of their greatness every day. Helen, who is so cherished and a darling, with a great memory and great ideas, says life is satisfying with a good cup of tea. "That's all I need," she says, "just a good cup of tea!"

Renee has a special way of communicating the depth of her feelings. She's the one who told me to hold her stuffed puppy toy when I was sharing a scary moment about being a little girl: I got lost at the Seattle World's Fair. Another day, when we were all singing and I was going around to check if everyone had the right page in the songbook, Renee was reading the words to the songs ahead of where we were. She looked up at me and said, "Isn't it something? Someone else feels emotions just like us." I am often struck with how much thinking does go on in the brains of these wonderful people.

Irvela will dictate what direction to take the class. She'll say to me, "I had a dream you were reading to us from your book." And I say, "Would you like me to read chapters of my book to the class as I am working on it?" She says, "Oh, yes." And I did.

Irvela's mother starved to death while taking care of her children during the war. Irvela was passed around for years to other relatives and aunts. One time, she ran away from home, hopped a freight train to California. Van Nuys, to be exact. She said her dad was called from his post in Washington DC to go find her. "How did he find you?" I was very curious.

"Oh," she chuckled. "There weren't too many young thirteen-year-old black girls in Van Nuys in those days. When my dad first saw me after his long search, he sank to his knees and cried. He thanked Jesus! I've stayed out here in Van Nuys ever since."

I find in working with these people that being loving and loving seems to be foremost on their minds. Somehow, the discomforts of living mean less than their focus on what's good and true. I find so many of these people kind, polite, caring. When someone takes time with them, that person is rewarded with their generous love and a great story, always a special moment to connect with. I feel our seniors, including the Alzheimer's patients, are a golden treasure. They are to be recognized not just for who they've been but also for what they still have to bring to us now. Look how much they have given to me. I have been sustained by their goodness.

When I am asked by my seniors or even the present baby boomers, "How do I stay young? Do I keep busy?" I always say it's not the busyness that matters; it's *what* you do that you feel excited and passionate about. Those who continue to have purpose and passion in their lives lead interesting, stimulating lives. Internally, they know they are valued individuals. What they do each day counts. They matter.

Statistically, many individuals die within six years of retirement. Maintaining self-worth eludes them. In recognizing your greatness, acknowledge the champion in you. Keep your passion, purpose, and health; we can continue to keep the joy and quality of our lives long into our senior years.

CHAPTER 12

Wisdom of the Ages

One of my favorite sites I frequented for over three years as a memory teacher is the Horizons. One day, the group focused on sharing special experiences in their life. Helen, had just celebrated her ninety-fourth birthday. I asked her what was her favorite birthday, and she answered, "Each one is the best." Helen couldn't see as well as she once did because of macular degeneration. Her hands were crippled from arthritis, yet her spirit and feeling of well being about herself is as good as anyone I've ever known.

In fact, she gave me a role model of high self-esteem, no matter what one's age or health. Life is a gift. She relished each present moment and each memory. She felt recognition through celebrating with her friends in the assisted living housing, and she also received phone calls from her friends back East.

In reflecting on Helen's wonderful attitude, I was curious about her early beginnings and asked her. She was born in New York. Her mother was a businesswoman and had a career. She didn't settle down and get married until she was forty which was very unusual in those days. One year later, when her mom was forty-one, Helen was born and was an only child.

She remembers sailing on the maiden voyage of the *SS Ile de France* when she was four years old. She said her mother sensed a beginning unrest in Germany in 1917 and felt it better that her family returns to the United States. Helen says what she remembers most was feeling sick on the boat.

This in turn triggered memories for the other participants in the group. Ruth, also in her nineties, told a story. She was one of thirteen children. The eleventh and twelfth of the brood were twins. When her mother came to America, her father was already in New York. She came across on the boat with her five young children. When she arrived at the docks, her youngest child, only three years old, had the measles, so they weren't allowed to leave the boat. Then another child contracted the chicken pox. She was quarantined at the docks for a month until they were finally allowed to leave the ship.

I enjoyed this group at the Horizons; they are seniors without memory problems. Many of them moved in after a spouse passed away.

I changed my teaching schedule at the Horizons so that I could have dinner with the residents after my class. Originally, I planned that each week I would sit at a different table so I could have intimate conversations with each person. But what happened was I sat at Helen's table along with Ruth who is ninety-three and May who is ninety-five. I never left.

Every week, I'd look forward to dinner with my girlfriends in their nineties. I am not sure what it is, but somehow the ninety-year-olds were the most happening, the most alert, the most vivacious; they had the most piss and vinegar. I asked them why. Ruth said it was because, "We've been through everything there is to go through in life, and we survived it."

Ruth shared how her husband died. "We were sitting down having our breakfast and chatting. When we'd finished, I got up to clean the dishes. I asked him a question, turned around. He was slumped down in his chair. I lifted his head but there wasn't any motion."

"What do you do in a moment like that?" I asked clumsily.

"What can you do?" Ruth replied. "You are in shock, just in shock. I tried to wake him. I called 911. The paramedics were there in minutes. They tried to revive him. They set him up in the ambulance and put the shocks on him, as they do on the TV shows. Finally, after two hours of trying to get his heart back, the doctor came out to talk to me. I told the doctor, it was okay. We had to let him go," Ruth continued.

"He was a wonderful man, so kind to everyone. I had been a teacher when I met him. It's a cute story. My sister lived in Pennsylvania. So, in the summers when I was off school, I'd go stay with my sister. I went to a party early in the summer, and we met. He walked me home the first night, and we were together the rest of the summer. Then I had to leave to go back to school and teach."

"So, did you write to each other?" I was curious.

"Oh, yes we wrote and kept in touch, but I still dated other boys."

"How long did this go on for?" Ruth really had my attention.

"Years." She laughed. "He worked at night in the summer so we'd have our weekends, and often, we'd go to the beach and make a picnic. It was fun. Then, I think it was the third summer. I was getting ready to go back to teach again when he said to me, 'Don't pack your bags to go back, just pack a light bag, because I have plans for us this weekend.'"

"Oh!" Ruth exclaimed.

"Yes," he said, "We are going to Las Vegas this weekend. We're going to get married."

"Just like that?" I asked.

"Yes." Ruth giggled as if it were yesterday. "And we went to Las Vegas. I never went back to my teaching job. I worked in Pennsylvania. Then when I retired, I worked with my husband in the hardware store business."

Helen winked. She was listening politely, although I think she had heard the story before. "That way she could keep an eye on him," she chuckled.

Then Helen wanted to tell her story too. Both women raved about their husbands, saying what good men they were and how great their marriages were.

I asked what made the secret of a happy marriage. Neither of them could answer except to say they really liked each other and respected each other. They continued to grow together and not apart.

Neither seemed to ever worry nor even consider infidelity nor not staying together until death do they part. It was a different time, they said. But truly, they kept saying how happy they were.

Ruth said, "There's not a day that goes by that I don't think of him or miss him." It had been eight years. But life goes on. I asked Ruth if she had children. "Sixteen nieces and nephews, I helped raise from all my siblings. I didn't want children. I see my nephews and nieces. They come to visit a lot. All my siblings are gone except for me." That was the first time her being alone and feeling it for a moment was apparent to me.

"How do you spend your days, Ruth?" I inquired.

"Oh, I am up early about 7:00 a.m. I take my shower, get dressed and come down for breakfast. I am so busy the entire day with activities. I do the exercise class every day at 10:00 a.m., and then we have another class. Whatever is on the board that day, I go to. Then we have lunch and the afternoon activities. After dinner, I may watch a little television with everyone. At 9:00 p.m., I get into bed and get out my book. I read until about 11:00 p.m. I read about three books a week. I love to read. I just don't have time to do it during the day."

Helen can't see because of her macular degeneration. Helen went on to tell me that she lived through encephalitis as a child. She had cancer in her ovaries and had a hysterectomy. She'd also had breast cancer and had a mastectomy. "Whatever they could take out they did." She said this with a smile.

Helen didn't behave like someone who couldn't see or someone who has suffered so much physically.

"Helen, you are amazing. How did you get such a healthy sense of self and self esteem?" I asked.

Helen didn't give it much thought. She said, "I guess I was just born with it." Then she said, "I was rather adored by my father, and my grandfather spoiled me terribly. I got lots of gifts and attention when I was little from my dad's customers, who used to give me toys. I always got attention from men." She smiled.

I look at Helen, I see her face. She has soft but wrinkled skin. She has deep blackheads up around the temple of her eyes. Her hands and fingers are terribly crooked from arthritis. Her back is a little hunched; she is always in back pain. She walks with a walker, and yet in my mind, she is beautiful. I think that's how Helen views herself.

She is teaching me the true experience of what it is to grow old gracefully. My Uncle Morris is also an example of that as well. As I write this in 2002, Morris is ninety-two and still working. He has a girlfriend, his toastmaster's weekly meetings in his home, and his concept therapy meetings. We just celebrated Morris's birthday in Las Vegas last February, and although he can't see as well as he used to, he is charming and caring and involved as he has always been.

One day, I asked my Horizons class what are the most prevalent memories in their lives. One couple that has been married for over sixty-two years just celebrated their daughters fiftieth birthday. What was so significant for them was they buried their first child during the Holocaust sixty years before. I asked the group what was most valuable to them.

Most of them discussed their happiness and satisfaction over careers or the fact they raised successful, happy children. Also, they have the love of their grandchildren. One woman said she almost felt guilty that she loved her grandchildren more easily than loving her own children. Then when she thought about it she said, "I have time to love my grandchildren. When I was raising my children, I had to work, raise them, and life was hard." She said that now she has the time to love them, just love them.

I came home feeling that maybe I was missing something in my own life. I don't have children and I've never been married. I was wondering if this emptiness I feel would always be with me.

Is it the love they had with their mate and then their offspring that made their love and life worthwhile? Was it what kept them going? They had a structure and commitment in which to make their lives continue and evolve. A few women had careers as singers, bookkeepers, or teachers. There were businesses for the men. They did it not only to keep their families going but also to enjoy their time of recognition and acknowledgment. I wonder, what continues to be purposeful when one's spouse is no longer alive, the career is extinguished, and the kids are all grown? Are grandchildren enough to keep going to want to live? What keeps the desire to live alive?

Attitude is one, diet is another, and love of something or someone else.

There is a book entitled *Where the Old are Young* where the same questions are asked. These are eighty to 100-year- olds living in Black Russia in the mountains named the Hunzas.

By employing these methods of memory with multisensory modalities, attitude, and diet with patients diagnosed with early Alzheimer's disease brings a new hope, utilizing those parts of the memory and visual abilities that are still intact. This assists the caregivers, the family and personal support systems, the medical support staffs, in stemming the prevention of Alzheimer's disease.

Scientists say that only 10 percent of the brain is ever used. If the unused parts of the brain can be stimulated (the mind is like a hologram), then access to information that has already been learned can also be recalled. Comparing the brain to a tree, we know that in the winter, leaves fall away, but in the spring new foliage, flowers, and fruits appear. The tree has knowledge of how to change the color of its leaves and create new foliage. By stimulating the brain, Alzheimer's disease could be likened to a winter tree, with the memory system assisting in sprouting new foliage and fruits. This could change our thinking about this disease from hopelessness to hopeful.

CHAPTER 13

Awareness When Your Loved One Is Slipping

My Uncle Morris began slipping at the age of ninety-two.

Instead of keeping everything in his life—his support groups, Toastmasters and Concept therapy, his girlfriend, his niece, me and his nephew, my brother and other long-term friends—all these were cut out of his life.

His sons' idea was to eliminate everything and everyone, then see how Morris did, later reintroducing things to determine what was still good and what caused him stress or discomfort. It's similar to finding out about food allergies; all food groups are ceased and slowly reintroduced.

The only problem with my Uncle Morris was that nothing and no one were reintroduced. He was slipping more. His word-finding processes became difficult, and he had a more difficult time speaking. He knew what he wanted to say, but it would come out as a stammer. Those around him—his caregiver, his secretary—often thought that meant he didn't know what was going on, that he was confused. I went to visit and found quite the opposite. He was very clear in his mind. He was very aware of his senses, his environment. He was sensitive to tone, to people's attitudes; he had great awareness. Why couldn't they see it as I could?

They weren't trained. They didn't know how to see what was still present but rather focused on what Morris had been in the past, which is unfair.

He still had a work schedule, although I don't know what he did exactly at the office, but many of his longtime friends said they would call him there. He had a workout bicycle; I was hoping that many of his tapes on motivation from great speakers over the last thirty years could be played for him to stimulate his old memories. This might be used as a positive retrieval method for brain stimulation and emotional revitalization.

Also, even though it was hard for him to speak, he could listen very well. I would call him and give him cheery news of the week and usually a good joke.

My uncle had been using a cane. He seemed to have a little limp when he walked. I was concerned. Many elders I've seen in the last few years are using walkers. When I ask them why they chose that over a cane, they tell me, "Oh, because it's so sturdy. It keeps me confident that I won't fall. It also has a little seat so that when I get tired, I can just turn around and sit down anywhere. It is just great."

I wanted this for my uncle as well. Many elders fall, and although they heal, they look like the purple people eater from the bruises. Some falls are more serious; someone can break a hip or shoulder—those are much harder to mend.

The tapes from Concept therapy and a chance for Morris to discuss and listen to a small group of friends or just one friend/family member is what I felt would be of benefit to him as well as keeping what worked in his life, friends, family, his lover, or activities. However, to stimulate more than one person I had to try different ways to stimulate a group. A medical doctor would not have this luxury to leave his office and intuitively figure out something for a group of his patients in their residential homes, which is why I had the good fortune as a teacher to do so. Yet in the coming years, I think medical doctors will begin to visit patients in their environments more so than before. A person's habitat can often show more about that person than by visiting a doctor in his or her office.

There are fun ways to stimulate the brain. Once, I brought in the movie *The Creature from the Black Lagoon* to play for my Alzheimer's seniors. It was just an experiment; they had asked for a scary movie. They were all excited, wanted popcorn, the lights low, wanted me near to squeeze my hand. They all became twelve-year-olds. Although that movie is a bit slow for our present sophisticated taste, they delighted in it. We played it one hour and then stopped and played the rest two days later.

When I was cuing them during discussion to recall scenes, they remembered. They had to be prompted, but once prompted, the recall was back clearly. This was the first time in three months that I noticed they could not only hold information for two days, but also recall it in their minds visually. Some even recalled through their emotions and what they sensed. I didn't know if they were recalling memories from when they had seen this film originally forty years before, or if it was new learning. Still, there was a tremendous stimulation, active participation, and emotional joy from this experience. So, I continued. Every few weeks, I'd bring in a film of their request. With each film, their recall was stimulated, and we'd discuss it. Anything from earlier than the 1950s was familiar to them, and it would ensure a conversation, and often, the participants would tell stories of themselves from that time.

I was fortunate enough to meet Sidney Poiter at a local Whole Foods. He was standing next to me in the checkout line. I burst out, "Oh, it's you! You're one of my very favorite actors, and you were my mom's too." He was handsome, slender, gentle, and kind.

"Thank you, and thank your mother, too," he said politely.

"Oh, she's dead," I blurted, "but I work with seniors now"

We chatted a few minutes. He said, "You are working with the golden group. They have all the wisdom and secrets in our society."

I said, "I know, I know, that's why I love working with them."

We smiled at each other and gave a nod-like bow goodbye.

The next day, I told my group about meeting Sidney Poitier. They cheered and asked if we could watch his movies, so the next week we watched *To Sir With Love* and talked about it. Then, they wanted to see *Guess Who's Coming to Dinner* and *Patch of Blue*. We entered into a discussion of those times, the early 1960s when racially mixed couples first came into growing awareness in our society. So, much of their recall is still available. It reminded me that people with Alzheimer's are still so very, very present and still have much to offer.

As I had mentioned earlier in this chapter about my uncle Morris, had he been able to continue his Concept therapy group classes on a weekly basis in his home, I feel the stimulation and camaraderie would have helped him cognitively and emotionally. His friends dearly loved and missed him, as I'm sure he missed their weekly visits. Sometimes, families make choices they think will support their parent, i.e. their loved one. However, as in this case, sadly their/his isolation from what fulfilled him lead to a lessening of his abilities.

CHAPTER 14

Treatments for Loved Ones

It's Sunday afternoon sometime between 1960 and 1970. I remember Aunt Flo would do her baking at that time; she would make oatmeal raisin or peanut butter cookies, apple strudel, or cinnamon rugela depending on her mood. She would organize and prepare for the week. Uncle Morris would read or listen to his tapes on Concept therapy or hypnosis and prepare for his business week. The children, Larry and Steve, would be out chasing girls, cars, motorcycles, or go- carts, depending on their age.

In my family, we were often bowling on a Sunday afternoon after we had a Chinese buffet at the Rickshaw in Tulsa. Gary and I mostly went to Sunday school, then a visit to our Grandma Mizel on my dad's side, before we went out for the Chinese buffet.

Many couples who shared with me those Sundays were in their special time, a family time of husbands and wives taking a walk in the neighborhood, listening to music, or reading a book by the fireplace, while the kids play outside with their dogs happy playing and barking along. It's usually a quiet, slow, relaxed day—one more free day before the week begins.

However, with Alzheimer's disease there are no free days anymore. Missing is the loved person that one grew to depend on, count on for little things, like remembering to bring in the mail, close the gate, call before leaving the office or run an errand to see if anything was needed before coming home—milk, eggs, paper towels. Those little things we come to rely on from another are rarely available now. Moreover, it is lonely, very lonely for both the caregivers and the Alzheimer's loved one. Lonely, yes, and uniquely different for both people.

The survivor's caregiver remembers the time reading and listening to music to look up to the other, and see his or her smile, wink, touch of the hand or arm, and feel comfort just knowing that the other is there—a life still filled with promise, hope, and years to still share together. Now, one looks up to see the look of the love, staring, sometimes blank.

It's lonely, scary, and painful. Still, somewhere inside the loved one there is a glimpse of cognizance. The spouse takes the little preciousness that is still there to hold on to, remembering that the spirit of the loved one is fully alive even if his or her mind isn't what it was.

This book is a tribute to those who have the illness, who still have something good in them. Yes, of course, the past will not be, but no one's life is as it was ten, twenty, thirty, forty, or fifty years ago. With all life comes change, some positive and some negative. There are many kinds of losses, each difficult, each with its unique challenges and rewards. This is another kind of loss. Yet, if you use the methods described in these pages—remember to use positive recall, look at those glimpses, and stay steady with what is, rather than what is not—there is more goodness to come. We can stimulate and nourish the memory and cells that are still alive, still functioning.

In the next few pages, I will lay out a generic plan for what to do at the beginning of Alzheimer's. Review this information with your health care provider.

I have received e-mails like this: "My mom was diagnosed with Alzheimer's nine days ago. She just turned sixty-two. I am not sure what to do or to think. My stepfather is in total denial, so there is no help from him. She just started Remilyn. She hates medicine, so making sure she takes it is key. I feel that my few friends are clueless to what this means now and will mean as this illness takes over my mom. I feel very alone and terrified. I work about seventy hours a week, but aside from my stepdad, I am all she has, and she is all I have. I talk to her every day. I cannot imagine that one day she may not know me. I am lost."

First, getting to a support group for the caregiver is paramount. Alzheimer's is a debilitating disease. One needs to not be alone. Personal therapy is also helpful in dealing with the flood of feelings that come into play. Once supports are in place, then one can begin an action plan to help keep what the loved one still has alive.

Dr. George Vinters who performs autopsies at UCLA says, "There are different reasons for cell death. However, in all cases the cells do not get enough oxygen and die."

Therefore, the logical thing to do would be to focus on keeping the body and mind oxygenated. You can get oxygen through breath, exercise, water, nutrients, foods, vitamins, and herbs that improve circulation.

This is a generic action plan. You, your family, your doctor, therapist, or caregiver can make it more specific for you in implementing these ideas. These ideas are for the patient; however these suggestions are good for everyone.

I. The first way we take in oxygen is through our breath.

Try ten to twenty minutes of deep breathing first thing in the morning. It is ideal to lie on the floor with a straight back, breathe in through the nose, and out through the mouth. Take the deepest inhalations as possible.

If breathing is a problem, there are excellent supports. There are pure oxygen treatments at local chiropractic or health clinics. If you can afford it, you can purchase an oxygen tube or have a machine set up in a bedroom. This allows pure oxygen to flow continuously in the room.

There is a profound method of getting oxygen by being in a hyperbaric chamber one hour at a time. This has very powerful effects. It is costly but helpful. In addition, if you do use this method, it is very important to do some memory training exercises immediately after the treatment, within the same hour. This way, the freshly stimulated neural branches have a chance to stay firmly rooted in the brain, rather than just taking in the new oxygen then letting it go out without being made use of. In the past, some researchers did not find hyperbaric treatments useful in improving brain function, but these studies did not include using mental or memory techniques immediately after the treatment. This makes a considerable difference in the effectiveness and usability of the oxygen treatment.

The body can also utilize oxygen by brisk aerobic exercise. A brisk two-mile walk every day or aerobic exercises for at least twenty to thirty minutes five times a week minimum is excellent to get the circulation pumping the blood throughout the entire body. If one is not able to walk, there are excellent chair exercises and videos that can support in one's daily exercise practice.

II. The water we drink is also very important for oxygen.

It is best to get purified water either bottled or use a special filter like Brita or buy a faucet attachment like Kangen alkaline water.

There are also drops one can buy to put into one's water to enhance oxygenation by seven times. The brain shrivels in older age because of dehydration; therefore, at least eight glasses of water a day prior to four in the afternoon is recommended. If you drink a lot of water in the evening, you may be up half the night going to the bathroom.

III. Food is also an excellent source of getting oxygen into your body. Fruits and vegetables are the best. Make sure you wash your fruits and vegetables in a special solution or vinegar to get the dirt and pesticides off *before* eating. Raw foods are recommended. Also fresh juices from a juicer will help to oxygenate your system. Wheat grass is also an excellent source of life food.

IV. Vitamins, herbs, and food supplements can also increase brainpower and circulate oxygen in the brain. 1,000 units of vitamin E daily (or more) are essential. Talk to your doctor.

Gota Kula herb is excellent. It is what elephants eat and they have excellent memories. Also, PS 100 Phosphatidylserine 100 mg and phosphatidylcholine are also recommended, one tablet in the morning and the other before bedtime. Choline and Inositol are important to improve memory and brain function. There is a book called *Smart Drugs* by Dr. Ward Dean, Steven Fowkes, and John Morenthaler that gives a lot of information about what to take to improve memory. Dr. Gary Small's *Memory Bible* is also a good source for recommended foods and nutritional supports.

V. Alternative Methods

Besides putting nutrients into our bodies, it is important to pull out toxic metals and poisons that can be hurting your system. A hair analysis is an excellent way to study what is happening in your body in terms of minerals and how your body is functioning. Most chiropractors or internists can do the test. It is better than blood and urine tests for fine-tuning what is happening in your body's tissues. This is a controversial test; however, in my personal experience, the results have been most helpful.

Besides herbs to pull out toxins, Chelation pills, or a Chelation drip can remove toxic metals from the system. (For Chelation therapy in your area, contact (800) 532-3688.) In addition, it is important to do natural liver and colon cleanses periodically. This way, your entire body has a chance to keep itself well and help itself heal.

When I had a serious car accident in 1999, I had quite a number of injuries including brain injury. I suffered with doctors who didn't know how to help me. Everyone joked, "The memory person lost her memory." Nevertheless, it was scary not being able to count on my mind for several years as I was healing. My brother said something important to me. He said, "Take notes. Remember what you are feeling because you've always taught memory in the past from a strong and healthy mind. Now, with your limitations and this injury, you'll know how your clients who are suffering from memory loss feel on the inside." What my brother said helped me feel I have the capacity to be an even better clinician because of these painful experiences. I will share what I did and then make some suggestions about what might be more appropriate for others.

I first went to see Dr. Timothy Binder at drtimbinder.com. Dr. Binder is a chiropractor, homeopathic naturopath, acupuncturist, and in my opinion, a genius. I had met him when I was in school in Boulder, Colorado, when I was eighteen and have been a patient of his ever since. A few months after my car accident, I could not multitask at all. I couldn't manage to do the laundry and pack a suitcase to get on the plane to see him. I had anxiety about planes. I was afraid I would crash. I called Dr. Binder; he soothed me, reassuring me that I would be safe getting on the plane and arriving to see him. I was. Immediately, he treated me with something called the balloon treatment. It is a cranial adjustment through the nose into the brain canal that opens up the areas that became blocked from the accident. Dr. Binder learned this from his teacher forty-five years ago. Very few doctors know how to do the procedure, but immediately after the treatment, I could begin to organize my thoughts.

Because the accident had caused such a trauma to my system, Dr. Binder prescribed Chelation treatments for me to boost my immune system. He increased my multivitamins and added more vitamins, including B complex, vitamin C, and a natural brain vitamin. He gave me a few hyperbaric oxygen treatments. I also had severe neck pain from the accident, along with disk herniations and bulges. I later got a TENS machine, an electrical stimulation machine that can help with pain that often physical therapists use in their treatments with patients, and used both acupuncture and physical therapy as prescribed by an orthopedic doctor. Therefore, with this combination, I was able to finish my studies for my master's degree.

I read Dr. Amen's book, *Change Your Brain, Change Your Life*. His book helped me understand what areas of my brain were affected and how my brain injury was affecting my emotions, which affected relationships with others. I was not able at that time to be as emotionally close, because much energy was tied up in just managing hour to hour to keep myself safe. After two years, I still was not quite up to par. Fortunately, I met Dr. Joseph Toomin and his wife, Dr. Marge Toomin. He was an engineer turned brain scientist, and he was able to pinpoint the problem caused by my accident: how I was hit, which part of my head suffered the trauma and injury. He suggested I get a SPECT scan to see where the injury actually was. From this scan, Dr. Toomin was able to pinpoint where my brain problem was, and then, he made a plan for me, which no one else at that point had been able to. I needed more oxygen in my brain. He said I needed to use my own memory system to teach groups of seniors, since I like them so much, love groups, and needed to practice my memory system more.

I continued with my writing class as a secure haven for expression and the forming and shaping of these chapters, and for psychological support as well as a personal psychotherapist which was a safe place to go to help me think and reclaim me.

In the few years when I was rewriting the book, another series of injuries happened. The monies I had spent fifteen years earning and saving to build a home for my future went into my treatments for recovery. I was left with nothing. My resources were depleted and my income was cut in half because I could only work part-time.

I fell and hit my head, causing more severe difficulty thinking, and it even affected my sight. I became farsighted from being nearsighted. My clavical was dislocated and more. I did immediately travel to see Dr. Binder who, yes, did the balloon treatment and the similar treatments as before. However, this injury was skeletal and permanent. There is no surgery I could find that was safe enough because the injured area is so close to the heart. To make matters worse, within two months after only three weeks of a school vacation, my boss sent me far away to drive to East Los Angeles, a commute that none of my doctors encouraged. In fact, I had written letter after letter explaining that the commute would further exhaust me and exacerbate my problems, and then the drive indeed caused new problems, compressed discs in my back, atrophy in my upper back and shoulder, and early osteoporosis in the area of my back, where prior I hadn't had back problems. The only thing that made me fight inside to keep my job and my will was to finish this book again with the new additional information.

After one and a half years of this suffering, finally the superintendent of schools had to step in to get me back to my home neighborhood to teach and get me off the harshness of the "ex-boss" who was causing emotional suffering professionally by asking me to do extra assignments and coming to watch me teach nine times in a four-month period. Most teachers are visited once a year or once every two years. I still did not have a boyfriend or soothing arms to comfort me, only the healing practitioners and my cats.

My brain's ability to function became so low, I could not organize myself, I was too tired to tackle duties outside of school, and finishing this project was just overwhelming. I could not find chapters I had written and had to once again rewrite the edits.

I moved to LA in 1996 to give myself a chance at acting in Hollywood. Because my brother and I are close, and we want to keep that connection, I fly to see him two to three times a year to be with him. It's just us; our parents are gone now.

In that visit of August 2011, I was able to secure an appointment with Dr. Eric Braverman. He did what is called a "BEAM" test on me. It confirmed my suspicions that my own mental abilities had been severely "used up" just in surviving others' unwillingness to be responsible for their actions and covering up their actions. I had to take on more than what I could handle, and it depleted me, all of me, brain, body, and finances. I had no energy to even teach a memory lesson to someone in need of me. That made me sad.

Dr. Braverman did a thorough blood test as well as tests from head to toe on every major organ and body part. What was insufficient in my body's ability to restore itself was pinpointed and addressed. Within one month, I took new brain meds, nutrients, and special hormones.

Therefore, within one month my energy was coming back. I visited a second time a month later. Dr. Braverman was concerned on one test on memory function I did not score in the uppermost ranges which for a memory expert is sad. I retested, and he came in to say hello to me and said, "You have an amazing memory." I was back!

With this new information, I add to the list of musts: Dr. Eric Braverman and his office in New York City Path Medical. Plan to spend the entire day. He is, I would say, another maverick and accurate in his ability to help patients recover themselves through his suggestions on diet, nutrition, and brain drugs. With his help, I finally could finish the book, organize myself, and return to an ability to function and get back to this matter, helping Alzheimer's patients get better, and give the caregivers their lives back.

PART 2

CHAPTER 15

Creating Your Life through Vision and Memory Methods

Here is an introduction to the memory system I use, a memory system so powerful it can increase memory abilities by at least three times. In certain tasks, memory will improve by as much as twenty times over the abilities you now have. The backbone of this system is "association."

An association takes two different pictures and makes a creative connection between them. You place one item on the left hand side and the other on the right, the same way we are taught to read and write in English. The two items are linked by an action verb ending in "ing," so that the two items are physically touching, physically interacting. The items are then linked—the first to the second, the second to the third, and so on. This is specifically the method of association used in my Brainsprouts memory training. Even in 400 BC, Aristotle stated, "Memory training is not only good for the memory but for the readiness of the mind."

There are three parts to memory: memorization, retention, and recall. Memorization occurs when we take in information and imprint it in our minds. Retention means maintaining the information, not losing or forgetting it. Recall happens when we look with our mind's eye and retrieve the information. The system of associating makes it easy for anyone to memorize information and recall it easily.

Thirty years ago, I was in graduate school at California School of Professional Psychology in La Jolla, California. I was curious why the memory system I learned from a then noted memory expert was easier and more powerful than others.

Dr. Mark Pezner, who was then an intern at California School of Professional Psychology, contacted me to say he was teaching a method of memory he had researched from an experimental psychology class; he invited me to come. While taking this class, many of my questions were answered. This is what I learned:

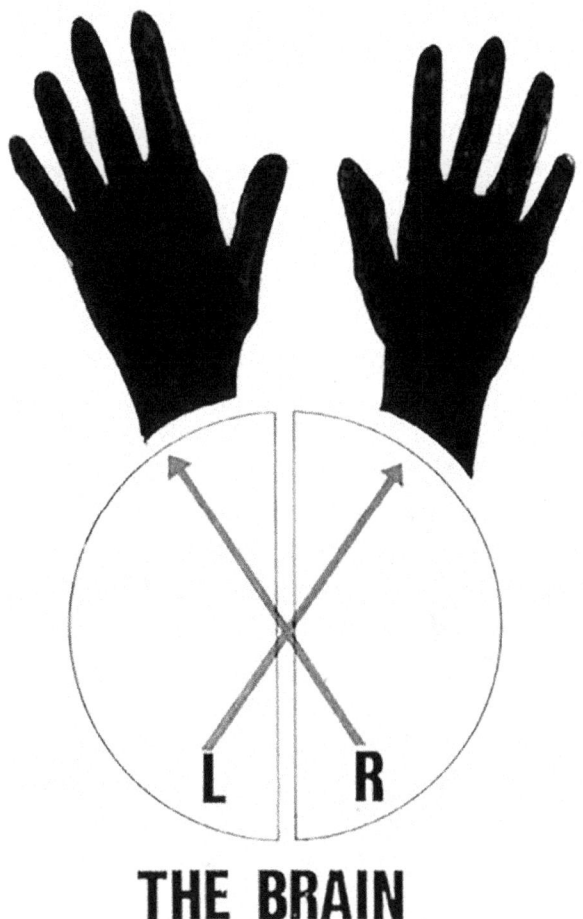

THE BRAIN

    Most of us know that there are two separate parts of the brain, the left and the right. The right side of the brain controls the left side of the body. The left side of the brain controls the right side of the body.
    To simplify, I will mention just three abilities of both the left and right sides of the brain. On the left is our verbal ability, our ability to speak. When one has had a stroke on the left side of the brain, it can inhibit speech. The right side is the opposite. It is nonverbal. This part of the brain recognizes facial expressions and body language.

Thinking is different, too. The left side of the brain involves logical thinking. The right sees and recognizes concrete or tangible intuitive information/pictures.

The brain operates with distinct differences in the use of time. The left side is the part of our mind that is aware of dates, appointments, and scheduling. It is also the part that wakes us at the same time every morning; if that is an ability you have or practice. Cats, dogs, birds—all animals have an internal clock that knows what time it is. The right side of the mind is oblivious to time. It operates when you are doing something you enjoy and are concentrating so that you are oblivious to time. We use the term "time got away from me." That can often happen while reading, painting, dining with friends, working on a project. Next time you are late say, "Oops, sorry. I was in my right mind."

As part of this experimental class at California School of Professional Psychology, I learned there was a study in which one hundred items were flashed on a screen at one-second intervals. Then there were also written words flashed in one- second intervals. What do you think the participants in the study were able to remember more, the picture or the written word? If you said the picture, you are correct. The participants remembered 75 percent more by viewing pictures than by seeing the written world.

Let's look at the distinctions:

They Can Still Remember To Love

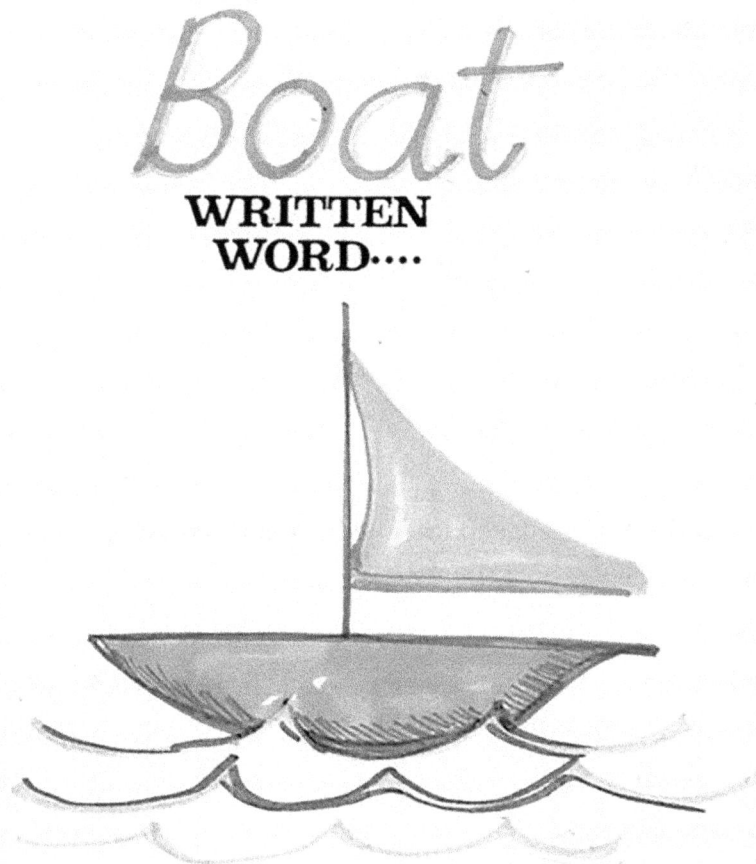

WRITTEN WORD....

VISUAL PICTURE OF WORD

Visual picture of the word. See the picture of the boat. (picture of the boat) What can you tell about it?

Now, imagine the written word "boat." What can we tell about it? It has two consonants, two vowels. It's in the English language.

Looking at the picture, people will describe the boat, the mast, the sail, and the water. There is a lot more information in the picture than there is in the written word. The mind retrieves information in the form of pictures more readily than any other form of information.

As an exercise for practice, imagine for a moment being on a boat. What are the things you would feel? You would feel the rocking and the wind. What would you taste? The salt in the sea air. You might touch the water, the smoothness of the boat. What would you see? You would see other boats, the shoreline, the seagulls.

What might you hear? The waves, the wind in the sails.

So, by seeing the picture in your mind you can access information from your senses. You could also take out a picture or draw a picture if you are not yet strong in your visual abilities. I didn't have strong visual abilities when I first started teaching this memory method. However, within eight months of daily practice, my visual abilities became very clear. Even my reading speed and comprehension improved.

This is very helpful because everyone has a different mode or style of learning. Some people are best at listening and learning, some at seeing, and some at touching. This way, no matter what a person's way of learning, a picture can access it. This can be quite a benefit when used for listening skills, presentation skills, and to enhance the effectiveness and timeliness of meetings.

◆◆◆◆ Three Types Of MEMORY

1. sensory

2. short —term

3. long—term

They Can Still Remember To Love

There are three types of memory. The first type is sensory. Sensory happens in just seconds. It's how we first learned as babies, by smell and by touch. The scent of a flower or scented oil is instant. However, the recall it evokes is stored.

Short-term memory is actually just thirty seconds. That is why people forget phone numbers and names so quickly. It's seven to thirty seconds, no matter what age. When someone says to me, "I have a bad short-term memory," I get upset because no one has a bad short-term memory. It is how short-term memory is designed: seven to thirty seconds. We might have an untrained memory—which is why the Brainsprouts memory system can help us train our memory.

Finally, there is long-term memory. How long do you think it works? It's forever; imagine seeing your first best friend in your mind. You can see him or her, or your mother, or your first pet if you had one. That's long-term memory. It's with you all of your life. The beauty of this system is that once you change a piece of information into a tangible picture, it changes from short—thirty seconds—into long term—forever, or as long as it is important to you. The beauty is that you make up your own pictures—no one else. This way you can remember what you need and recall it when you need it with immediate ease.

visual
in

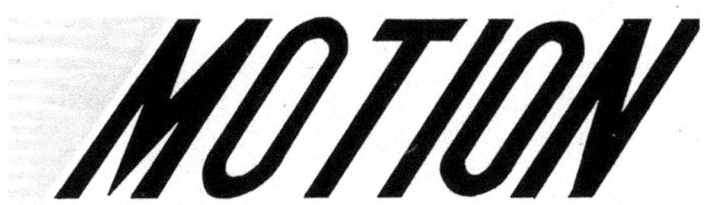

unusual

When people were asked what helps them to be able to remember something, they all found that if something is visual, unusual and in motion, it helps them recall. There is a famous animated Disney movie, *Fantasia*. In it is a scene where Mickey Mouse is "The Sorcerer's Apprentice." There are brooms carrying pails of water. Anyone who has seen it remembers it no matter how many years it has been.

If you didn't see *Fantasia*, think of your favorite cartoons, Bugs Bunny, Mighty Mouse, the Road Runner. When you recall this, does a picture come up in the screen of your mind's eye? It's good if it does. This is as simple and easy as the memory system gets. You ask a question, and the picture comes up on your mental screen.

In the experimental psychology class, four different pictures of a piano and cigar were presented.

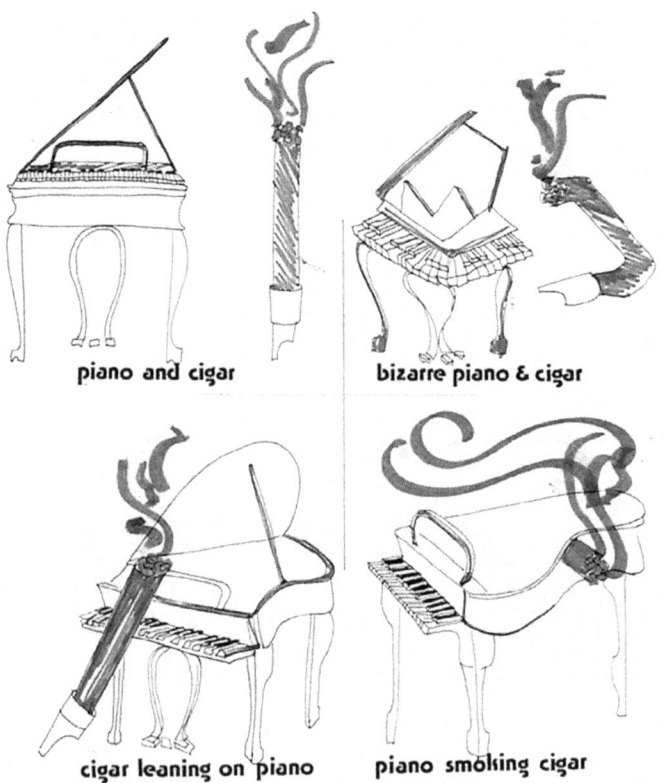

The four pictures were: the regular piano and cigar; the bizarre piano and cigar; the cigar leaning on the piano; and the piano smoking the cigar. Of these four pictures, which is the easiest for you to recall?

Most people say the piano smoking the cigar. Usually, they look at each one, but the piano smoking the cigar is the one that most people remember most easily. Let's look at the distinctions. The top two pictures are separate. They are not touching in any way. The bottom two pictures are two pictures as one. They are connected.

In picture three, the two items are linked by a passive verb "leaning." The fourth picture, the piano smoking a cigar uses an action verb. They are directly interacting and touching. This is the picture that most people remembered most often. Action verbs are "hugging, kissing, squeezing, jumping into, rolling over, clapping, cutting, etc." Notice that this picture is also easiest to recall because it's visual, unusual, and in motion.

This leads us to how and why this Brainsprouts creative memory system works so powerfully and effectively. It connects two items using an action verb ending in "ing." This is the way the mind naturally recalls.

The Creative Power System

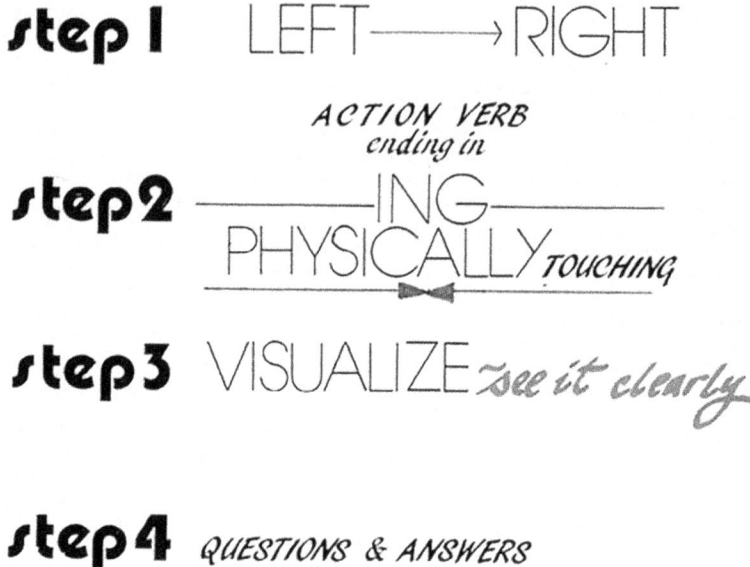

This is a four-step process. You place one item that you will be associating on the left and the other on the right. The same way we read in English, from left to write.
Step 1 Left to right
Step 2 Action verb ending in "ing"
Step 3 Visualize—see it clearly in your mind's eye.
Step 4 Questions and answers

As in the picture of the piano with the cigar, there are two items touching each other. The piano is smiling. That is an action. Then we see it in our mind's eye. To recall it, we ask, "What was the piano doing?" We see it smoking a cigar.

It is important that you visualize the image in step 3 clearly; otherwise, it will be difficult for you to recall the association when you need it. It is also important that when you recall and ask the question, that you "re-see" the image. This way you are seeing. You are not actually memorizing. If you don't see it and try to memorize it, you will not recall it as effectively. You must see the picture in your mind's eye, and you must see it again for recall.

Otherwise, you are practicing a different memory system in which you have to repeat everything over and over and over again by rote. Then you haven't learned anything new or new ways to improve and help yourself.

Now, let's take a simple example to review. Just to make sure you have the steps down properly.

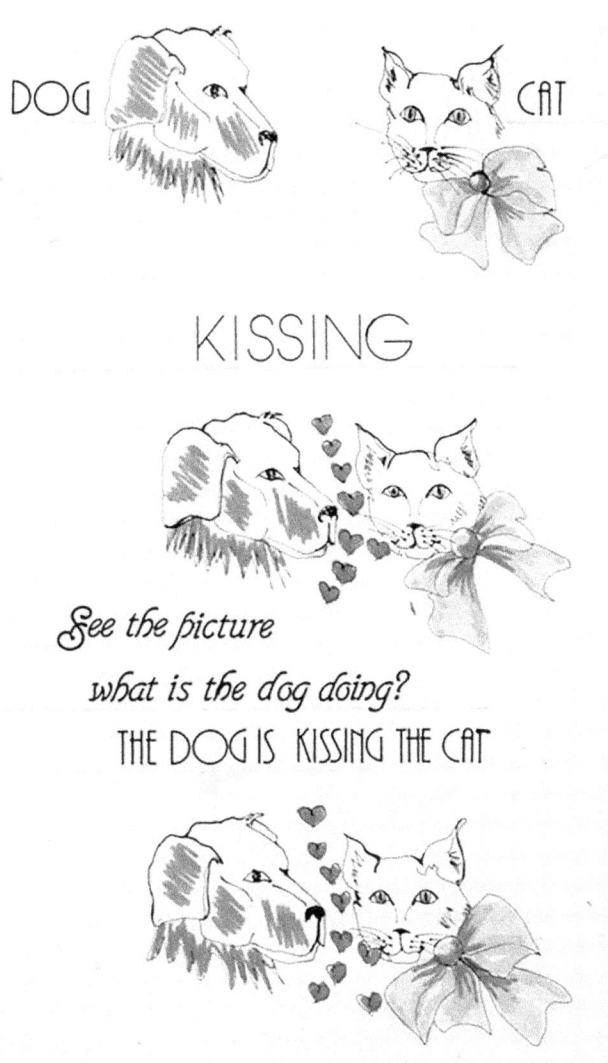

Imagine you see a dog and a cat. The dog can be any kind of dog—your dog, a neighbor's dog, a stuffed dog—and a cat, any kind of cat. What can you see the dog doing to the cat? Someone will say chasing or barking. "Chasing" is an action verb. Yes, it ends in "ing," but are the images physically touching? No, they are not. So, this would not make a good association with "barking," again you have an action verb that ends in "ing," but again, the images are not touching. "Carrying" works. "Snuggling together" works, but remember you want them doing an action together. "Playing together" works.

Make sure when you ask the question, "What is the dog doing?" You are then re-seeing the picture of a dog and a cat. You do not want to memorize the picture. You want to see it.

Now, let's say you have to go to the bank. For a picture of the bank, visualize money. Now, move the dog out of the picture on the left and replace it with a picture of the cat. This is how to associate lists.

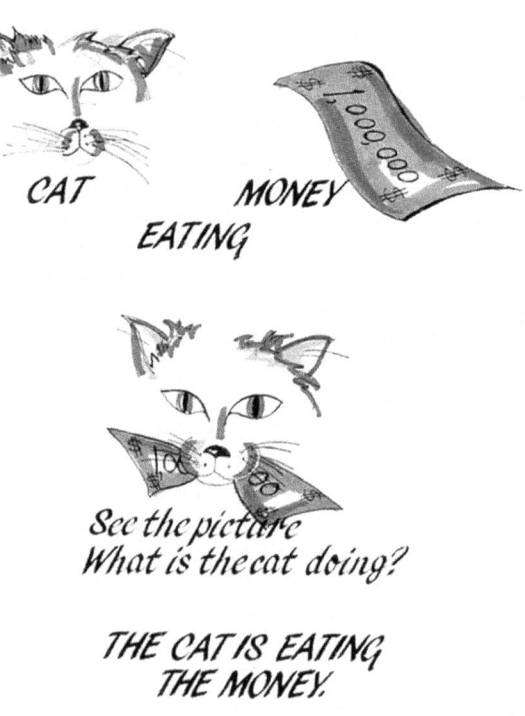

Imagine the cat is on the left, and the money is on the right. What can you image the cat doing to the money? Eating. The cat is eating the money. If you say playing with or counting the money, this is good. If more than these two items are included, it is not accurate. Remember, you can only memorize two pictures at a time. The dog to the cat. The cat to the money, and so on.

I am showing the linking of 1) Left to right 2) Link the two items by an action verb ending in "ing" where the items are physically touching and interacting. 3) Visualize and "see" the image and action occurring, and 4) The recall is through using questions and answers. What is the dog doing? You see the picture of the dog playing with the cat or licking the cat. It is in the recall or re-seeing the picture that causes the synapse to fire and release neurons. This is what stimulates the mind and increases neural foliage in the brain. This is what improves brain function and increases memory capacity. This method of associating pictures is very good exercise for the brain.

Pictures can also be used for motivation and achieving goals. When the mind sees a picture, it has a place to focus. For money, you could see hundred dollar bills, a Rolls Royce, a mansion. For time, you can see a clock, an hourglass, or a grandfather clock. For good communication, you can see a telephone or a happy family communicating. For a good relationship, two people shaking hands, kissing, or sharing a meal together by candlelight.

Begin a list of your own using tangible images and then link each item to the next using an action verb that ends in "ing." Make sure to use a different action verb for each association. Also, link the items only as two pictures at a time.

Start with yourself. For instance:

1. Me action verb ending in "ing"	2. item
1. I am <u>bouncing</u>	2. an egg (poached, scrambled, and so on)
2. The egg is <u>riding</u>	3. a bicycle.
3. The bicycle is <u>carrying</u>	4. the trash.
4. The trash is <u>taking</u>	5. his vitamins.
5. The vitamin bottle is <u>making</u>	6. the bed
6. The bed is <u>washing</u>	7. the floor
7. The floor is <u>eating</u>	8. an apple

Double check the pictures in your mind's eye to make sure you have one item on the left and the second item on the right, and that the action is occurring from left to right. Make sure they are touching, and you are only associating two items at a time. When you recall the list, ask yourself the question, "What is the item on the left doing?" You should see the picture come to your mind's eye. Continue asking the same question for each of the numbered items in a sequence until you have finished the list. These are excellent brain training exercises. If you make a list every day and associate the pictures, even for just five to ten minutes a day, it will increase the neural foliage in your brain. Thus, this will increase your cognitive and mental capacities. That is why I call this method "Brainsprouts". This is what guards against mental decline from lack of use or depression.

It took me an hour to learn this the first time. Then, it took twenty minutes to make my own list. After a few times, it took me ten minutes, then eight, then five. By the ninth time, I could memorize a ten-item list in two minutes. Each time you recall the picture, you are making new neural branches in your brain.

Each time you scan your mind to come up with a picture, you are stimulating the brain. When you make the association of the two items in your mind and then "re-see" the picture to recall the information, it causes the synapse to get excited. Then, it fires, releasing more neurons. Those neurons form an architectural scaffold and create new neural branch growth from the existing live cells. So, if Dr. Carl Sagan, as mentioned in chapter 2, is correct, each time one fires the synapse, it releases ten thousand new neurons. That means when you are using this Brainsprouts memory system, you are making tens of thousands of new brain cells from the existing live cells. It does not take much effort, once you learn it and practice it regularly.

The results of remembering is profound which is why I've used it for the last thirty years with students from kindergarten to seniors, in colleges, with business people such as CEOs, with actors, Alzheimer's patients, stroke patients, and even brain-injured people, including myself. All have improved with time and practice.

The Sounds-like Method Makes Information Tangible

Now, we move into the sounds-like method. The sounds-like turns an intangible piece of information—a word, idea, or concept, into a visual picture. Here's the first example of the sounds-like.

Heart rate

See a heart and a rate. Make a % sign. Again, see the heart linked to an action verb "jumping" from left to right. See the heart jumping on the rate.

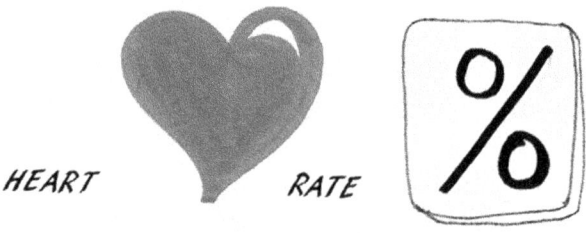

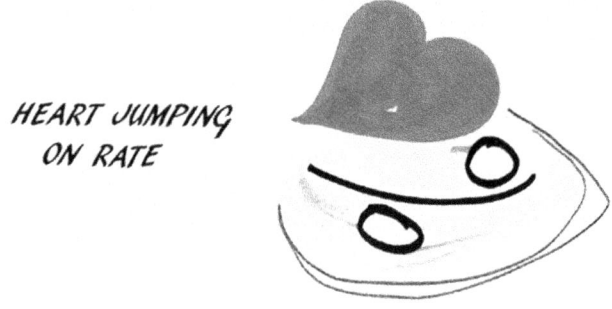

Discount

What does "dis" remind us of? It could be a disk, a record disk, or a computer disc. "Count" might remind us of numbers 1, 2, 3. So we can see the disk knocking over the numbers. This also gives us the definition of discount—lowering the price.

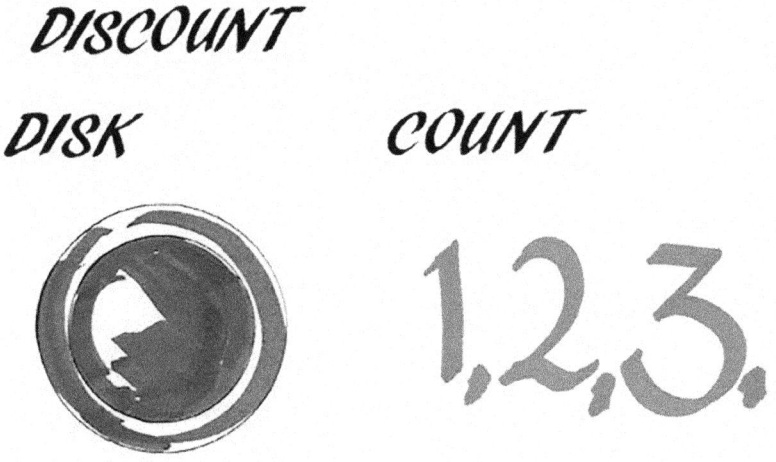

DISK KNOCKING DOWN NUMBERS

Organism

An organ, we can see, but an "ism" is nothing, so we can free-associate and come up with a prism. Here we see an organ smashing a prism.

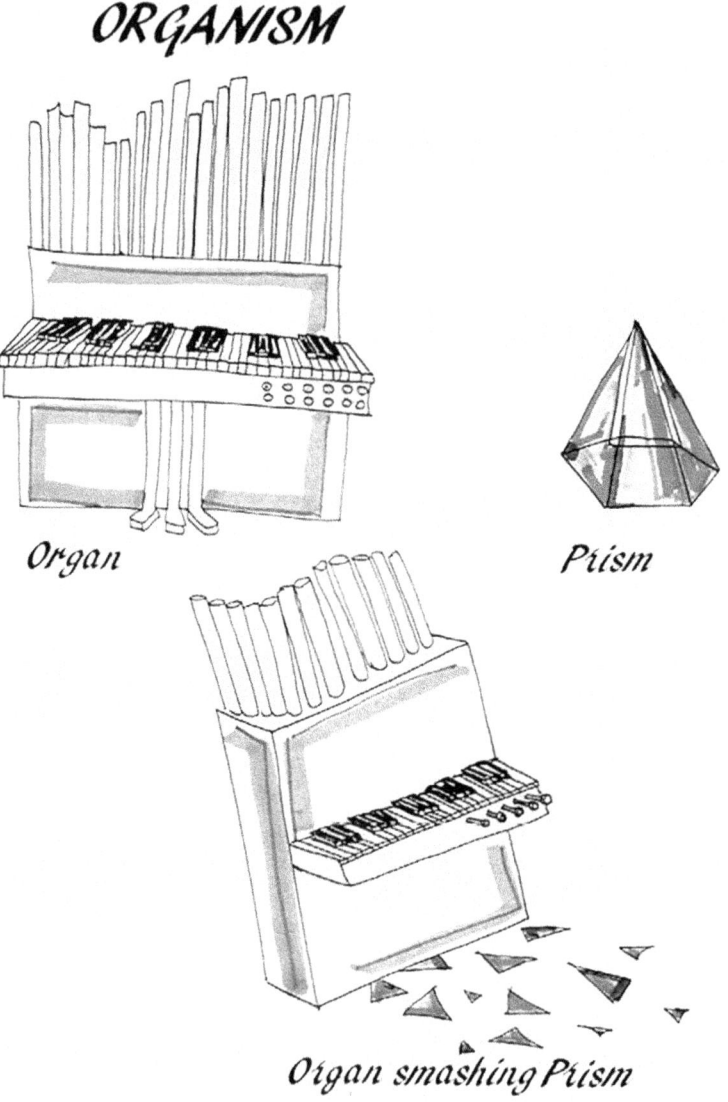

These are examples of ways to turn information into tangible pictures in order to associate information. From here, it is easier to remember information because, again, you are changing it from short-term memory into long-term memory. The mind encodes information in the form of pictures more readily than other information.

You can use my techniques to recall large amounts of information. Also, you can help your loved one remember information more easily by making the information tangible. Then, you can help your loved one remember not just the picture but feelings, colors, and sounds. This helps the picture stand out, which also makes recall easier. With these methods, you cue yourself by asking questions and then seeing the answers as the picture. Remember, you ask the question, "What is the item on the left doing to the item on the right?" An Alzheimer's patient or stroke victim will not be able to cue himself or herself. You will have to do that for him or her. However, if you take the time to teach them to think in the language of pictures, the recall will come more easily. It will help communication between the two of you. It will also help the Alzheimer's patients feel more relaxed, more comfortable, and more in control. It will make you feel better too.

Vicki Mizel, Brainsprouts, 2003 update

I was teaching in nine different assisted living facilities two hours at a time. This is why I have the research. Doctors usually see their patients in their offices. Rarely would a doctor be able to spend eighteen hours a week with patients in their own living environments. I only used a control group and a memory training group at two of the facilities.

The two groups, Sunrise and then Marriott, are the early cognitive groups and one Alzheimer's. I spent four weeks with the Marriott doing other things for stimulation rather than memory association. With Sunrise, we worked with associations early on. What I have found so far is that the rapport is wonderful either way, and the ability to learn names using effective methods of association works with a small familiar number of about eight people. Yet, if another five new names are introduced that are unfamiliar, it befuddles the person who had great confidence earlier in remembering the eight names.

The Sunrise group was able to increase not only associations of lists but names much more effectively from the combination of association and other forms of stimulation. Also, even the Alzheimer's people had great fun with images and found them "far out" and laughable.

One thing that made me quite happy was what the activity director Sharon at Sunrise on Topanga said to me: "With your program, none of my Alzheimer's patients have deteriorated mentally. You can see, however, they have gone down physically." It's apparent by the lack of more serious exercise.

I really didn't know when I asked her. I thought perhaps it was just adjusting to the environment and making new friends. But Sharon affirmed to me that the program did help them.

Also, a woman, Edith, who resides at the Horizons, who happens to be the sister-in-law of a gentleman, Oscar, said to me a month or so ago: "I can see Oscar is getting better."

These are definite indications to me that this is more than just my hope. I have actual witnesses of improvements that are noticeable to a regular eye.

Also, there are medical codes under a doctor's prescription that now are accepted by some insurance companies to cover "cognitive rehabilitation therapy." Perhaps both individuals and groups could have that available to them. Dr. Arnold Bresky of Camarillo, California, was the first medical doctor I know of who was willing to implement this for his patients.

CHAPTER 16

Follow Your Dreams

I was going through some of my boxes from storage and came across a box labeled, "Pre-Vicki Memorabilia." Being curious, I opened the brown cardboard box. Inside were pages yellowed from age. A newspaper dated 1944 contained obituaries of those soldiers killed in action both in the army and navy. At the top of the newspaper was a beautiful picture of my mother in a lavish white gown with a caption: "The Current Girl of the 24th Signal Heavy Construction Battalion at Camp Murphy, Fla." Pfc. Harry Waxman entered her photo in a camp contest. *A sophomore at Milwaukee State Teacher's College, Miss Berg sings and dances at clubs and parties to help finance her education. She is a graduate of Riverside High School.*

I had never known my mom went to a teacher's college. I thought she'd gone to business school.

Also in the box was an old program of *The Belle of Baghdad*, with a caricature of my mom as a harem girl on the front cover. I opened the playbill. On page one were the scenes and the synopsis of the story. On page two was a list of the cast of characters. My mother's name, Harriett Berg, was listed as the lead, "*Jewel, his favorite daughter.*" I saw inscriptions from her classmates saying,

"*Dear Harriet, The best of luck to a sweet co-monitor. I am so glad I got to know you because you are a real sweet girl.*"

"*Boy, that last kiss is sure going to be a blooming thing.*"
Walter Shapiro

"*Well, Harriet, long will I envy ... after this is 'Carmen.'*" Tom Leonard

"*To the Lead. Good luck, kiddo. You're really great. (Keep up your voice work!)*" Aileen Hall

"*It's been grand being in this operetta with you and hope we can do it again.*" Dori Mac Donald

"*Dear Harriet, Everyone enjoys your clear voice and acting.*" Sincerely, Mac Smith

"*It's been lots of fun. You were an ideal partner. Lots of luck.*" Tom Leonard

I had never seen these items before. I was perplexed. She had so much promise.

My mother was talented and beautiful. After two years of college, she had to drop out to work to help her family. A year later, she moved to Chicago at the age of nineteen, where she lived with a roommate and sang in clubs.

I remember hearing the story of how she and Daddy met. He was visiting his friend, Harry Miller, who was married to my mom's first cousin, Charlotte Tugenberg. Harry and Charlotte lived across the street from my Aunt Flo and Uncle Morris, my dad's brother. Daddy was in the living room where he and Harry were talking business. He saw the picture of my mom as the "Current Girl." For him, it was love at first sight. He pursued her long distance, at first, in Chicago. After many more months of singing lessons, my mother moved to Los Angeles with her family in hopes of breaking into the movies. She was twenty-two. "I want to be a movie star," she told her mom and dad. "I want to be like Maureen O' Hara and dance and sing in the movies. I had all the leads in all the plays and operettas in high school. Mother, it's my destiny. I can do this. I want to do this," she pleaded.

"My shenna velt. My beautiful world, duchta, my daughter," her mother replied, "since you were in diapers I had hoped you'd become a famous movie star or marry someone rich."

My dad visited her in Los Angeles and took her to Fox studios to talk to someone there. I think it was one of his army buddies. My mother was told, "Nice girls don't belong in the movie business."

After several months in Los Angeles, my dad got tired of the long distance relationship: sending flowers, paying an army buddy to write her beautiful love letters (which she thought he'd written). He proposed one night over the phone.

My mom asked if she could call him back. She told her mother of his proposal, Grandma Ida said, "We have been poor your whole life, and we are still struggling here. Sammy just made an offer to marry you. He has money from oil wells. He'd be able to take care of you and us too. How can you turn that down for a wish? You haven't even found anyone to give you a screen test," her mother said doubtfully.

"We came this far from Milwaukee. We made it through the Depression," my mother said, looking for some encouragement, although she felt she couldn't risk the opportunity for her parents to be taken care of and finally have an easier life.

My mother was torn. She really wanted to give herself a chance in Hollywood, but she also felt the burden of her parent's early losses of their parents in the war in Europe. My grandma and grandpa both left their parents for America at an early age, never to see them again. They were poor, very poor. For years, my mother and her brother, my Uncle Bob, had to take the streetcar to the Tugenberg Bakery to get day-old bread and donuts to eat. Grandpa was a furrier and a shoeshiner and later a baker as well, but during the Depression, times were tough.

My mom called my dad back, "Okay," she said. "I'll marry you." She told me years later that when she hung up the phone from that conversation she sat down and sobbed. She was heartbroken later to find that it wasn't he who wrote the love letters and that she married someone who couldn't express his love.

Many, many years later, the morning before my mother's funeral, my dad and I were sitting on his bed, talking. We both had our heads bowed. I asked him, "When did you stop loving Mommy? (They divorced when I was fifteen years old.) Daddy answered quickly, "I never did stop loving her." I couldn't believe my ears. Why didn't he fight for her, try harder to give her the emotional connectedness she needed? I turned to him.

"I didn't know that, Daddy. Maybe she didn't even know."

He said, "I told her to do whatever she needed, just don't leave me."

"I didn't know that either, Dad."

Then, he paused and said, "There's one thing she never forgave me for."

"What's was that, Daddy?"

"I promised her before we got married that I would buy her a hall for an evening, so that she could sing to a full audience on stage. She'd asked me several times through the years."

"Why didn't you do it?" He could afford it.

"I thought when she'd make elaborate meals and have friends over for dinner then sing to them afterwards, she was fulfilled. I guess I didn't feel renting a hall was really that important." My dad spoke in a low tone. "Now, she's dead." I wonder if he felt perhaps she'd been happier had he given her room to do what she loved on her own terms. I think I wondered, too, and still do.

He didn't get it, never really did. She cooked gourmet meals almost nightly, kept a beautiful clean home, and made us all breakfast almost every morning: pancakes, waffles, French toast, and eggs. Daddy got a homemade lunch to take to work daily. All she wanted was a chance to perform, a chance to be seen. In her mind, she gave up an acting career, or at least something in the area of performance, to be appreciated as a loving wife and mother. Yet, I remember a particular time when Mom and I were watching an old classic movie on television. Maureen O'Hara was starring. At the commercial, Mom looked up teary-eyed and said to me, "That could have been me!" And it could have been; we'll never know.

But this I do know. When you give up on your dream, you give up on a part of your life. My mom never fulfilled a valuable aspect of her talent. If she had? Well, perhaps her marriage would have had a better chance. I would have a role model of a woman who chooses her own well-being first, rather than taking care of everyone else and leaving herself last.

My mother's choice to give up singing to marry my dad, Sam, had a profound effect on the rest of her life. This decision was ultimately a financial choice to please her parents. Many of us make decisions based on finances and survival rather than our true desire to work with our gifts. We all have a special gift that we are destined to give as a contribution to society. If we do not honor this intrinsic desire, bring it forth, perhaps we are not fulfilling our life's true purpose. Deepak Chopra has many quotes in his book, *The Seven Spiritual Laws of Success*, to help us accept the present moment.

We all have life lessons and choices. This is what I learned from my mother: Always do what makes your heart sing. When I was a teenager, after I had my first job as a Miss Pure Magic Makeup salesgirl, I gave some consideration to future work. "How do you know what job is the right career?" I asked my mother.

She answered, "Because you love it so much you'd do it whether you got paid for it or not."

In my initial work with Alzheimer's patients after my mom died, the work was my own antidote to depression. The welcoming faces of the elders gave me a safe place to be, to express myself. This reminded me of the happiness I had as a child with my grandparents. I also realized that teaching and training in memory has been my way to reduce the risks of my getting the illness. I have followed my fate. Although I don't wish misery, loss, and this kind of emotional pain on anyone, something good has come from it for me. I have a career now, helping others through this memory system along with my other programs to assist new passion and purpose in our lives. We all at some point have to pick up the pieces of a broken life, a broken heart, or a broken spirit. This is how my own spirit was healed.

Years later, in 1988, when I had my first diagnosis of Epstein-Barr, I couldn't work at the pace I had for years before, traveling, giving seminars, speaking engagements. I, too, became heartbroken. I was about to give up my beautiful home in La Jolla. My health was poor. I was truly scared. I had already thought about moving to New York, for I had enjoyed my business trips there since 1985. The author of many Dale Carnegie books, Arthur Pell, said to me during a meeting we had in Manhattan, "Can you use your memory system to create a new life, using visual pictures?" I thought about it and answered, "Yes."

I decided to begin with myself as a guinea pig. I created new goals for myself using pictures of what I wanted: an apartment with a Manhattan skyline, dance classes, acting auditions, art openings, someone to love and share it all with.

Having worked with the memory system since 1980, by 1989 my mental prowess became so fertile that it demanded to be free. I had to try activities that I had wanted to be part of since I was a child. I wanted to dance, play, sing on stage. I wanted to paint with oils, take acting classes, and perform in movies, plays and television. I no longer wanted to write any business proposals or wear business suits for a year.

I made my pictures of the "end result" I wanted to create. I wrote what I wanted the accomplishments to look like, feel like, smell like, and what emotions I wanted to feel. I was willing to give up everything—a La Jolla condo, a Baby Benz 190, the ocean because it became clear to me that I needed to move to New York. The Upper West Side was my preference. I made the decision and committed to it.

Three days after this decision, I was invited to a tea party in Los Angeles. As I entered the room, I announced, "I need to move to New York, and I need a one-bedroom on the Upper West side for $500.00 a month." Within seconds, a woman, Lisa, approached me. "I don't know if this will work or not," she said, "but my renters just gave me notice. If you will take this apartment sight unseen and pay rent this month, it's yours."

I called my brother to ask his opinion. He said, "Vicki, I love you, and I value you as my friend and my sister. However, you will be even more valuable to me if you live in New York." That was so he could visit and stay with me. I called Lisa and said I would take the apartment. I sold some jewelry that week so I could send her the money. That was March of 1989. In May, I moved into what I called my "miracle apartment" in New York City.

Not only did I create a dream I had for myself but also was able, over time, to regain my health. Thus, my new brainchild was born. I created a seminar, "Passion Quest: Finding the Work You Love and Loving the Work You Do."

CHAPTER 17

Passion Quest—Never Too Old

I was in the UPS store in Toluca Lake, California. From the PA system, the song "Aquarius" was playing. Images came back to me of the play *Hair*. My family went to Las Vegas in 1968, and my Grandma Ida came to join us from Los Angeles. It would mean so much to Grandma to be with us, my mom said, so Grandma came. The MGM had *Hair* playing; I wanted to go. Grandma was my date. I remember the lines, "let the sun shine, let the sun shine in, the sun … shine in …" when the naked members of the cast came out, and Grandma was dying in her seat. "Duchta, Oy, Ooy, Vehzmer." Her face turned white, then pink with embarrassment; she hid her eyes with her hands. I was laughing and enjoying the music.

When the baby boomers are living in assisted living residences at the age of eighty, I can see them, too, recalling the days of the stage play *Hair*. It was in the heart of the revolutionary days of Berkeley: sit-ins, walk-ins, tear gas, marches, the Peace Movement, LSD, Vietnam, and Maharishi Mahesh Yogi.

We live longer now, so the sixty-year-olds of today are still young, and there are many more years of enjoyment to be had. The biggest reason (aside from illness, accidents, and improper nutrition) for atrophy in one's mind or one's body is lack of use. If you sat on the couch for three days and didn't move and fed yourself messages such as, "You're too old. You're not enough. You're not good enough," how do you think this would make you feel? Not great, huh. This is what we tend to do to ourselves. There is no reason why any of us should stop what we love to do just because our age has changed.

Many retired people are starting second or third careers. The Art Student's League in New York City is filled with happy, retired people living a passion that had been dormant for years. One assistant principal who had taught music for thirty years retired at fifty-five and became such a great sculptor that no one believed he hadn't been sculpting previously. He told me quietly, "I made love to a lot of women in my youth." Apparently, he had quite a touch also in wood and in stone.

George Burns, a true role model, was still performing in his nineties. He had contracted to work in Las Vegas from the age of ninety-five to one hundred. He celebrated his hundredth birthday in 1996 and still made television appearances up until his death.

It is important to know that at any age we can always make new pictures and new passion. It makes a difference in our lives at any age to keep ourselves in activities that we love. This is the secret of a long, fulfilling life.

Dr. L. Stephen Coles, MD, PhD, Department of Surgery for UCLA, has been doing a study on centenarians. He found what is in common with all of them is that "they all desire to have something to do, and they all have a reason to get up in the morning. Whatever they like to do as a hobby is very important to them, and they do it." They all had a variety of interests but they were all intrinsically motivated. He said, "They were so busy it was hard to schedule them to sit down for an interview with me!"

If you knew it was possible to change the course of your life in the time it takes to read this chapter and complete the questions and follow through with the assignment, would you be willing to? The contents of this chapter can help change your life at any age. They provide a way to create a safe space within yourself to remember what made you happy at play as a child, what nourishes and supports your well-being, what you see as your greatest accomplishments. From reviewing your answers, insights come firsthand, helping you decide what you feel passionate about. Then, you will create a vision of what you would want to do if you could wave a magic wand and have a new career, a new life. You must give up doubt, fear, and other people's opinions. These instructions are paramount while you are doing the exercises. If you knew that you would be successful at whatever you wanted, would that make it easier for you to get started right away? Yes!

There is a saying in Russia, which is also in the Bible: "Where there is no vision, the people perish." In Minsk, Bella Russe, the people rebuilt the city from the rubble after World War II. They had no money. They worked all day in the factories, yet at night, they often went with very little sleep to rebuild the city. Within three years, the city was rebuilt. Today, Minsk is one of the most beautiful cities in all of Bella Russe.

Passion Quest is a program about discovering your precious gift and making it your life's work. The process we will be using in these pages is as follows: remembering, discovering, or rediscovering the dream that is yours. Then, you will make a specific action plan to achieve your desired results.

Many people awaken each morning without energy, drive, or verve. Also, our external structures are crumbling through corporate downsizing, shifts, and the death of spouses, illness, family conflicts, or feelings of abandonment.

Not being able to count on what we've been used to for security creates uncertainty. We often hear negative comments from people important to us—spouses, children, relatives, friends, parents, teachers—too often. We listen to them instead of to ourselves. We listen to their voices so much that our own inner voice becomes faint, and even if we hear it, we no longer trust it. Our choices become restricted because our own self-imposed doubts and fears limit our thinking. Through experience, we know that if our creative desire is not being met, we cannot be happy.

That is truly the beauty and the struggle of the spirit of being human. We seek to satisfy our souls.

As a memory trainer, I've worked with pictures for the last twenty-five years. The pictures were used to create goals and remember names, lists, speeches, and scripts. Teaching classes and imparting this knowledge to others, I found myself, as well as my students, becoming more powerful in creating and achieving goals. I envisioned trying to employ my memory system with stroke patients; the next week, a friend asked if I would work with her mother who just had a stroke. Her mother improved dramatically within three weeks. Independent of each other, both the physical therapist and the speech therapist asked me what I was doing because she was improving so quickly.

Another example: When I wanted to work with Alzheimer's patients, within a few months the dean at San Diego Community College hired me. Later, a research study through UCSD was implemented. I was amazed at the power of mentally focusing on the "end result." I took a class called DMA (direct mind access). One exercise was to write what you wanted, then ask yourself: If you could have it, would you receive it? If your answer was yes, then you visualized it coming true. I visualized myself in a circle with Alzheimer's patients, showing them how to remember names and list of tangible items. A few weeks later, a boyfriend of mine at the time, handed me a card and said, "I fixed a copy machine today over at UCSD. I mentioned your desire to work with Alzheimer's patients. The doctor gave me his card and asked for you to contact him."

Students of mine using the system were achieving goals. One woman sold her home in a market where little was selling. She got the agent, the title person, and herself to all visualize seeing the sale happen within one month. One month to the date, her house was sold. Another man got himself out of debt after just working with me for a day, writing down his goals and seeing the end result achieved. Now, he teaches a course called "Debt-Free," using the power of pictures and focusing desired results. We all knew that something more than just memory was going on, but we didn't know exactly what. I learned it was the power of pictures, along with feeling the feelings of the *end result* that was making such dramatic changes possible in my students' lives. Again, once you have created your vision, refocus on it and truly claim it.

Still, we can't always be happy. However, choices and determination make a difference in accepting circumstances. I went back to the Horizons where I had worked for three years. One of my Monday night table-mates, Betty, the only one still alive, told me her story. She had a heart attack and had been in the hospital for six months. "They almost lost me," she said. "It cost my insurance and Medicare one million dollars to save my life, but look at me." She showed me a flat belly that had once been round. "Look, no hands. I have exercised, and now I don't even walk with my cane. (She does keep it with her for she needs to use it a little but not as dependent as she had been as before.) The doctors call me the "Walking Miracle."

"I am impressed, Betty." I congratulated her and gave her a kiss on the cheek. But even more, I was curious. "Betty, did you decide to get well because a million bucks had been spent on you?"

"No, that wasn't the reason. I have my children, my grandchildren, and my great grandchildren. I am vital to their lives." And with that, she picked up her cane, then steadily but slowly walked to the dining room on her own. "Are you coming in?" she asked. I followed behind her.

As I walked in the dining room and looked around, many faces I once remembered were no longer there; no longer alive. Mickey, a blond woman in her eighties who usually had her meals with her husband, was wearing a fashionable round hat. She had two caregivers with her. I slowly walked to the caregiver first and said, "Where's Marty—her husband? Is he dead?" Mildred, a beautiful Asian twenty-year-old said, "Yes." I turned to Mickey, who was eating, and said to her. "I am sorry, I am so sorry for your loss." She nodded to me, still chomping on her sandwich. This time, her eyes looked dull; grief was present, very present. Mickey had been a violinist in the New York Philharmonic when ten years ago a stroke left her unable to play. She had always been at my classes except when she was in physical therapy. She was gracious and smiling, which had impressed me. But this day, even I wondered. "How is she managing?" Only her children now, and caregivers, and no lifelong companion. I wondered if Mildred was on an antidepressant. After all she's been through and all she's continued to strive for, sometimes life just gives us too many hits, and we get a setback. But knowing Mickey, she may sleep a little more now, but she still had a good appetite for that sandwich.

Psychotherapists and psychiatrists have discovered that our personalities are formed from the ages of zero to six. The Passion Quest Program is comprised of four major questions. The first one is, "When you were five years old, what did you want to do when you grew up?" This poignantly explores early desires. When we are children at play, we gravitate to our natural desires and instincts. Play gives rise to qualities, abilities, talents, and interests. An opera singer I know was already singing as a child. A bank president's favorite game was monopoly.

What makes a person happy is different from one person to the next. For instance, actors and speakers tend to love recognition and audience dynamics. Others may be terrified of being in the public eye and are happy behind the scenes, tucked away somewhere.

Get a pad of paper and a pen and get ready to go through the Passion Quest process.

What did you want to become when you grew up, and what are your earliest, happiest memories?

Feeling *safe* inside is key for the participant. These exercises should be done in a comfortable and relaxed setting. Nice music or some form of meditation might also help to unlock these powerful memories.

These questions at this stage are designed *not to focus on career* but on experiences and moments that are genuine and happy. This will help later in getting to what supports and satisfies feelings of well-being.

What experiences make you feel most at home within yourself?

An Australian actor and hands-on healer spoke to me once about his childhood. His father wanted him to be a car mechanic. He tried to please his father but finally realized he was not pleasing himself. He quit and began an acting career. The first time he was on stage, he said, "I loved it! I felt like this was home!"

This question focuses on what you do to make yourself feel nurtured in your own special way: splashing in the ocean, hiking in the hills, walking on the beach, boating, playing on a computer, reading a book, making love; whatever is right for the individual.

The kind of activities one chooses to relax, renew and enjoy oneself speak volumes about the person because the activities that nurture a person support his or her well-being. For now, it is important not to focus on career but on what makes one feel good.

This exercise addresses the internal make-up of the individual. Fred Love, the animator who created Fred Flintstone, said he was lucky. "I always loved to draw. When I was sixteen, someone at Disney told me they'd pay me to draw. I have flown all over the world and been treated wonderfully doing what I love the most."

A young animator who just got his first job at Disney has a different story. As a child and even now, he watches cartoons. He always wanted to be an animator at Disney. When his best friend got a job at Disney, he was invited in as a temporary assistant. He met all the right people; within six months he was a full-time animator. I asked him, "What got you the job—who you knew or your vision?" He said, "The vision led me to meeting the right people."

As you think about what makes you feel most at home within yourself, you will become more comfortable with exploring and answering these questions. A pattern will begin to take form and become a roadmap. As you analyze your road map, your direction will be revealed.

What are your greatest accomplishments to date?

This question is pertinent for any age. This can be a significant accomplishment or recognition by others. "What are your greatest accomplishments to date?" The question answers internal needs that feed the individual emotionally.

Accomplishments might include recovering from a chronic illness or critical disease, making money, supporting oneself, or even returning to school. A multimillionaire who had been unhappy in his marriage got enough courage to separate and divorce his childhood sweetheart and wife of thirty years. Everyone has achieved major accomplishments. It is important to recall, acknowledge, and list them. One woman took stock of her accomplishments, looked up at me and said, "I'm amazing. I have accomplished some very noteworthy tasks." Immediately, she began to feel better about herself because she remembered who she was. It is important not to get down on yourself when circumstances are less than favorable. Remembering your abilities and accomplishments can assist in spring-boarding you back to confidence, self-esteem, and trusting your strengths once again. This is especially pertinent for older workers or for housewives who want to enter the job market for the first time. Also, visual techniques must be included to help improve self-confidence and focus.

What are your identifying patterns and needs?

We have asked four major questions to gather information that is pertinent to the individual. Now armed with this information, see what has become most apparent to you about yourself. What are your needs? What are the things that support your well-being? What are the themes and patterns that you have discovered or identified about yourself?

Although everyone's individual pattern of success is unique to each individual, I have discovered four things that are critical to my ability to be successful. First, I need one person in my corner, a true and trusting confidant who is there for me no matter what. Second, I need an audience. I need to share, to be able to give, and to be received in that giving and be given back to. Via this shared experience, we uncover new awareness as in the chapter where I learned with the Alzheimer's patients what made them stop their lives emotionally: New ideas, and approaches, develop because of the group experience. Third, I need a certain amount of physical exercise and alone time to be "on my own," thinking, creating, inventing, processing. I need a beautiful and quiet space to come home to, preferably with a loved one and definitely with a furry, loving animal, a dog or cat.

Last, I work best on a project with a definite break after the project is completed. I need break time to wind down, recharge, debrief, and have room to create the next phase or project. I think we are all the same in that we have a positive self who works at optimum levels when we receive our core needs. We have counterproductive ways of behaving and feeling when we don't get what we need.

Please take a moment and reread the previous questions. Think through what you have written for your answers. It is time to evaluate and see what has become most apparent to you about yourself. It is important to identify and list these items and make sure they are given full attention and merit.

From these exercises, past participants have discovered aspects of themselves that have often been missed in a therapist's office. These are powerful tools to bring insight for oneself. One woman had been in therapy for six years, but something was revealed in the Passion Quest program that she had never discovered before, involving her relationship with her sister. Later, this insight helped her resolve a conflict with her supervisor; her entire career and life became more positive.

It is important that all exercises are written in as much detail as possible. These writings should be first impulses and first impressions, with no holds barred. Besides feelings of delight and joy, sadness and anxiety are common feelings. It is important to allow whatever comes.

Now you have all the ingredients necessary to go to the exercise that you've been waiting for. "If you could wave a magic wand, what would you truly want to do? *Create the picture!*"

CHAPTER 18

If You Could Wave the Magic Wand—Creating Your Vision!

If God, the fairy godmother, or a genie appeared and said to you, "I am so proud of you. I've watched you, seen your goodness, and I want to reward you. I'm going to give you whatever you want, the existence you have always dreamed of. You, however, must tell me what it is as specifically and in as much detail as possible, then I will bring it forth for you to receive. You need to be very clear."

If someone wants to give you something, tell him or her exactly what you want. For example, say you'd like a bicycle. Just any bike won't do. You must specify what make, model, color, speed, and extras. That way, you will receive exactly what you want.

All the previous exercises have been a preparation for this moment, to state the true desires of your heart and say "yes" to them. Often, we will shut down within ourselves because we believe we are too old or just not lucky enough. But for the purpose of this exercise, you must be willing to accept that what you want is a viable possibility. If you could wish upon a star and wave the magic wand to do whatever you wish independent of time, money, circumstances, and other people's opinions or judgments, what do you truly wish to do in your heart? What is the picture of your ideal life or career?

Now, I want you to draw a picture of the end result.

(Drawing is important, even if stick figures are your specialty.) The picture is powerful because the mind needs a focus. Once the focus is clear, the unconscious knows no time boundary. This enables the unconscious to think the goals already exist so it acts as if it is happening right now. To make this picture even more specific and real, bring in all of your senses to the picture.

These action steps are what you must do to bring forth your vision. First, write down all of the feelings that you would want to experience in your ideal life or career. Describe the feelings in the present tense using all of the five senses: hearing, tasting, touching, seeing, and smelling. Write it all down exactly as you would like it to occur. (Even if you think it's far-fetched, go with it.)

When I was acting in New York, I saw a picture of the end result. I was on stage; I was speaking the lines truthfully and so affected that honest tears rolled down my cheeks. I felt exhausted and exhilarated. Then I'd see the audience. Tears were streaming down their cheeks; I had touched them, too. I visualized it and felt it over and over. Then one night many, many months later when I was performing at the Actor's Institute in a one-act play called *The Little Box* that moment what I had envisioned was realized. I played a character who had accidentally killed her parents driving in a rainstorm. They told her to pull over, and she told them, "Not to worry." The lines went: "The next thing I saw was the doctor's face. He told me everything would be okay. How could he lie to me like that!" The brother in this fantasy scene (my character killed herself that day, the anniversary of her parents' death) said, "I don't blame you, no one blames you."

And my character's line was, "Why didn't you tell me that before!" The tears were streaming down my face as if I could have lived had I not felt shunned and guilty, had this brother spoken up. After the scene, I went backstage and peeked through the curtain. I could see the audience. Many had Kleenex's out, and some were wiping their cheeks. I did it! This is the moment I visualized.

Now, it might have been helpful had I also envisioned an agent coming backstage to sign me, envisioned a contract for a movie or television series. But we live and learn to make our visions. What I do know is that my visualization came true, and many more desires have come true since then. Not everything has come about. Some things we don't understand. My teacher, Dr. Roger Bruce Lane of the Cosmos Tree in New York City, says to put it in the Light of the Most High for the Highest Good and tell yourself to let it go. I feel we need to trust we receive that which is best for our learning.

I worked with an older widower who felt very alone. He drew a picture of himself dancing on a cruise ship, sailing the high seas, surrounded by lovely ladies. He then envisioned having dinner for two in his home with a new love in his life. Although he didn't meet his love on the cruise, the action of taking the cruise gave him room in his mind to dream of what he wished for. Within a short time, he remarried to a dear friend of thirty years who became widowed too.

Another woman, Ruth, a widow, missed the companionship of her husband and friends but also didn't want to give up her home. She worked out a compromise: She moved into an assisted living residence for two months at a time, and then her daughter would go to San Francisco and get her to stay in her house for two months. This way, she was very happy and had the best of both worlds.

After these steps of writing and drawing, the next step is the improvisation of acting as if what you've envisioned is already achieved. Create this as a scene the way an actor would. Even if you don't act, it's fine to just go with it—it's fun. You can write out on a piece of paper a day in the **LIFE** of your vision of your new life, step by step throughout the day beginning from when you first wake up, until you go to sleep at the end of the day. You can use other people in the class to participate in your vision and do an improvisation of a particular scene. An improvisation is when you just "make up" something. For example, if you visualize being a teacher, classmates can be your students asking you questions after you "improvise" giving a lecture or an assignment. If you want to be a newscaster you can see yourself on television delivering the news. Imagine being an investment banker with your name on the door of a big firm, and you are closing deals on the phone or in person.

This exercise will bring forth the internal experience of having the goal accomplished. This way, you already feel that you own the experience in your body. You are no longer wishing, waiting, or hoping for it to come. After this exercise is completed and the feeling is brought into the present, the next step is to truly commit to this goal and focus on it. Then, you must create five action steps to bring forth the vision in reality.

A simple example is this: You want your ideal weight to be (145 or whatever yours would be), and right now, you are 156. First, you see yourself at the weight of 145, seeing your sleek new figure on the scale which says 145.

1. Write down the five action steps.
2. Decide to lose weight.
3. Make a deadline by which to have the weight lost.
4. See a picture of yourself at that weight.
5. Make yourself a recording to play to reinforce your desire.

Only allow foods that support your goal in your home.

The next exercise is to see each step already completed in your mind.

> Step 1. Daily exercise for thirty minutes (see yourself on an exercise bike)
> Step 2. See the scale at that produced weight goal.
> Step 3. Drink eight full glasses of water (see an empty Sparkletts bottle)
> Step 4. Put a picture of your present face on a body or your body at the desired weight or see yourself in the mirror with your skinny clothes.
> Step 5. See yourself listening to your recording daily. (It is suggested to reinforce your goal twenty-one times a day for forty days to create a new habit.).

Whatever images you make for yourself, make sure you see those steps clearly in your mind. See the end result already accomplished. Keep practicing it. Seeing it in your mind alleviates potential fear, anxiety, and reduces procrastination. Most negative feelings are a result of a past experience. When you envision what you want to create in the future, it assists you in overcoming resistant feelings. It empowers you to get going and create the good that is awaiting you. Once these steps have been taken in your mind, it is easier to bring them forth into your physical life.

Sometimes, a vision does not come at first. In this case, going from the "inside out" is fine. This means writing down your feelings and values first, then allowing the vision to come from there. Many times, participants will still suppress the goal they really want because of the voice that says, "It's just not practical." At this moment, remember to go with the true desires in your heart. If it makes you feel more comfortable, you can also make a secondary vision as a backup plan. Do not shortchange yourself. Give free rein to your imagination. As you spend time on your dream, your vision gets clearer.

Once you have your picture of the end result you want to create, your written design of your new life or career and your emotions, feelings, qualities, and values, it's time to implement your action plan. Make sure that your vision is in a place where you can see it several times a day.

Begin taking the action steps that you wrote to support your vision. Recognize that any type of change is often scary and uncomfortable. That is why many people stay in unhappy or miserable circumstances. At least, the situation is familiar. Also, unhappiness takes on a certain comfort, and then it becomes frightening to change because of the energy it takes to get out of the inertia.

1. There is still no guarantee that the change will be better. However, usually when you shake things up, something new will occur which will be better. Yet, often a person will wait until there is a major occurrence or upset to make a change—such as an injury on the job, an altercation

with the boss or another associate. There may also be loss, illness, or death. Whatever moves you to make the change, when you have decided to do it, then you must adopt a solid action plan. Here are the steps:

2. Decide to change. Until there is a decision, circumstances will continue as they have been.
3. Take the necessary action to do this.
4. Put the vision—drawing that you created in a place where you can see it. Also, review the internal feelings you want to experience.
5. Your mind needs a direction in which to move and create energy. As long as you vacillate, it will be difficult to feel energetic and directed. For example: One Passion Quest participant told me prior to the class that he was listless, lacked energy, had quit exercising and doing the things that he had once enjoyed. Once he made a commitment to embrace what he loved to do, he was feeling much better. He also began an exercise program, regained his energy and resumed bicycling with his wife. (Something they had both previously enjoyed doing.) His action step for this was to "see" himself on his bicycle. He could feel the wind on his face, the movement in his legs and felt the joy in his heart sharing the activity of bicycling (or pedaling) with his wife on her bicycle too.
6. Work your action plan. Review your five action steps and work on at least one each day. As you complete one step and get it accomplished, add another. Acknowledge yourself for each step that you have accomplished.
7. Exercise. No matter what you are going through in your life, at least twenty minutes of some exercise each day that makes you sweat will improve your overall feeling of well-being. It is also important to keep up good nutrition including vitamin supplements. Abstain from any form of recreational drugs, alcohol, or excessive sugars.

8. Experiment with finding out what doesn't work for you. This is important in the process. With clarity, you can pinpoint what you want and continue to write and envision it.
    Do not compromise. Be true to yourself.
    If you are not happy with yourself in a situation, you will not be able to make it last.
    One man took a job as a CPA because his dad said he would have to make a living and support his family. This man loved designing and building. Yet at forty-two, after being a CPA, a CEO, and a CFO, he was so unhappy, he quit. Now, he feels it's too late to go to engineering school; he is really having a hard time. He resents his children because he sees them as bills he has to pay. He sees his wife as someone nagging him to do what he dislikes so that the family can stay in the lifestyle they are accustomed to. He would like to build a tree house, but he has to find a job. Does that sound familiar?
9. Review the question, what makes you feel at home within yourself, and what makes you feel most happy and accomplished? This may help you pinpoint what you need to have in your environment so that you can make a lateral shift before making a complete shift.
10. Say *yes* to *yourself*. "Y" stands for yielding. Everyone is going their own way and will try to persuade you to go in their direction instead of the one you have chosen. Yield the right of way and continue on your own. "E" stands for encouragement. Remember the little engine that could. "I think I can. I think I can." This little engine continued until it knew it could, and it did make it. "S" stands for support. Everyone needs support and a support system. No one can do it on his/her own. Round up the troops. Tell people what you need, ask them how they can best support you and how you can support them. The book *Team Works* by Barbara Shear gives very good suggestions on creating a support team. Also, there are many networking groups available.

11. Keep at it until you achieve your desired goal. The only way not to achieve your goal is to quit. Eventually, whatever you want will come to you. In the book, *Think and Grow Rich*, Earl Nightingale says, "Whatever you ardently desire, strongly image and fervently act toward, you will achieve!"
Practice your vision daily and keep the faith!
A perfect example of this is the movie *Hoop Dreams*.
Two students of similar age, upbringing, and income were picked to be groomed to make it to the NBA. One student was able to get money and a scholarship. The other student, ineligible for the scholarship, had to transfer to a worse school with a less favorable team. His father was a drug addict who went straight for a while and then relapsed. His mother was motivated and became a nurse.

The student who received the money and scholarship had an injury and eventually quit the game. The student who had the hardships ended up making it in the NBA despite his personal setbacks. When he was interviewed, said he always saw himself playing in the NBA. This vision never left his mind. He was committed to it and never wavered, no matter what.

12. Keep at it until you achieve your goal. Persistence is key. A friend said to me one time, "Don't quit, because if you do, someone else will get what you want." Keep practicing your exercises. Review the five basic questions. Clarify your perfect life including feelings, qualities, and values. See the vision in your mind. Read your written descriptions and see the vision daily. Imagine this happening to you. Imagine scenes in your mind of yourself in this new role. Fantasize this life at different times of the day. See yourself in the morning, afternoon, and evening: What activities are you involved in, or how you are preparing for the day? Act as if you are already there in each scene.

Speak in positive terms. Always assume it is going to happen. If you expect it, it will come. Anticipate already having your accomplishment in your life as opposed to waiting for it to happen. There are some great examples of this in Catherine Ponder's book *Pray and Grow Rich.*

Ten years ago, before Susan Rabin, the author of the book *How to Flirt, Date and Meet Your Mate,* was a writer, she took a mini-Passion Quest course. She was still working for the Board of Education in New York as a counselor and was deciding whether to quit, start her own business, or to stay until retirement. She also wanted to write a book, but she just wasn't sure what to do. Later that day, we were in a deli having lunch. I said, "Let's act as if you've already published the book. You're on talk shows. Someone is coming up to ask for your autograph." There were others at the table with us. I got up and asked Susan for her autograph—praising her book and her courses. Susan signed; we all laughed uproariously. Today, Susan has completed her second book. She has been on all the big talk shows and holds classes on a monthly basis at Stand Up New York. Yes, of course it takes hard work and determination, but the vision helps to guide your course. Once you follow these twelve steps, you will succeed at your vision.

Sometimes just the insight derived from going through this process is enough. It doesn't necessarily mean that you must give up on your present life or career. Adding activities to one's life can be meaningful and often times just as important. During one Passion Quest course at the University of Tulsa, a participant, Nomi Beale, realized that she loved to go skiing with her husband in Vail, Colorado. What became clear to her was the importance of buying their own place so they could ski all winter. This enhanced her life so much she was content to stay in her present position, earning the money to buy the winter residence.

Another person, Eric, from a Passion Quest class in New York at the Learning Annex knew he couldn't give up his job just yet. But he gained so much insight about himself and felt so much happier that his job performance improved and he sold four times what he had previously.

When what is important in one's life is identified, then it can easily be added as a component to be appreciated and enjoyed.

CONCLUSION

When I began writing this book my purpose was to solely focus on Alzheimer's patients. I wanted to offer support to those struggling with a decrease in cognitive abilities using memory training techniques and to further explore various factors that may lead to one developing the illness. Improving ways of communicating by cuing and anchoring in images can help family members, care givers and the medical practitioners in relationship with the patients. All of which are essential for holistic care and increasing chances of improvement.

    However, upon completing the book, as I looked through my own life and themes that played out in this desire to share my findings for both prevention and improvement I found a greater component of this book. Rather a companion within the same book, a new application for this work began to appear to me. I began to see the possibilities for this book to exceed my original goal of helping Alzheimer's patients and their families improve a difficult condition, to train the public and the baby boomers generation to keep their emotional, spiritual and physical health into the centenarian ages. I began to realize these methods and research could also support anyone through their "black hole" and re-emerge with renewed passion, purpose and vision.

    I recognize themes and patterns in my own life and the life of my mother, and grandmother. These women lost themselves and/

or their dreams because they didn't know how to get out of their "lost self", because of loss of a mate, or "lost self" because of giving up a life long dream.

In analyzing my own work and stories, I see how I wanted to change my destiny of the feminine in my family (1) to identify and claim who I am as a person independent of a partner, (2) to stay true to life long dreams I'd envisioned for myself, and (3) to hold firm to my beliefs and claim that which I knew to be true even if the outside world or research to date thought differently. For example, in 1984 I knew that the brain could regenerate, and now thirty-one years later medical science confirms this to be true. However, the findings were not confirmed when I first experienced that knowledge when I worked with my Alzheimer's patients.

I have had my share of bumps in the road and difficulty, as have we all, and I was blessed, truly blessed with great love and affection, warmth and security as a child that has helped me, (with a lot of support), hold on to me. Through the later years of family loss through death, divorce, illness, and then my own tragedies; I was able to pull through. I believe that strength in my will and heart is because of what had been given to me, put into me by goodness from my grandparents, aunts, uncles, parents, my brother, and closest friends and medical confidants. This book is really a sharing of experiences of stories, lessons, and techniques. It is an experiential program to aid the progression of whatever is one's heartfelt destiny. At each stage in one's life, this book offers advice on (1) how to examine it, (2) how to learn from it, and (3) how to fill in the gaps through new learning; giving oneself, memory training, and a way to recreate a new vision. This vision could also be a dream that has been either lost, left behind, pushed aside, or never begun. Passion Quest offers methods or techniques to gain the internal and external supports and pinpoint what one needs to remain whole and a complete self no matter what age we are or what challenge we may be experiencing.

So it is my privilege to share significant life changing experiences of my life, my Uncle Bob's life, my Grandma Ida, my mother Harriett, my students and clients, and the beloved

Alzheimer's patients I have had the pleasure of working with. I learned of the human spirit on this sixteen- year journey of developing and writing this book.

I hope that you can glean something from these pages to assist you in continuing your life with the capability to receive everything you've ever wanted. As my Uncle Morris would say, "Carry on".

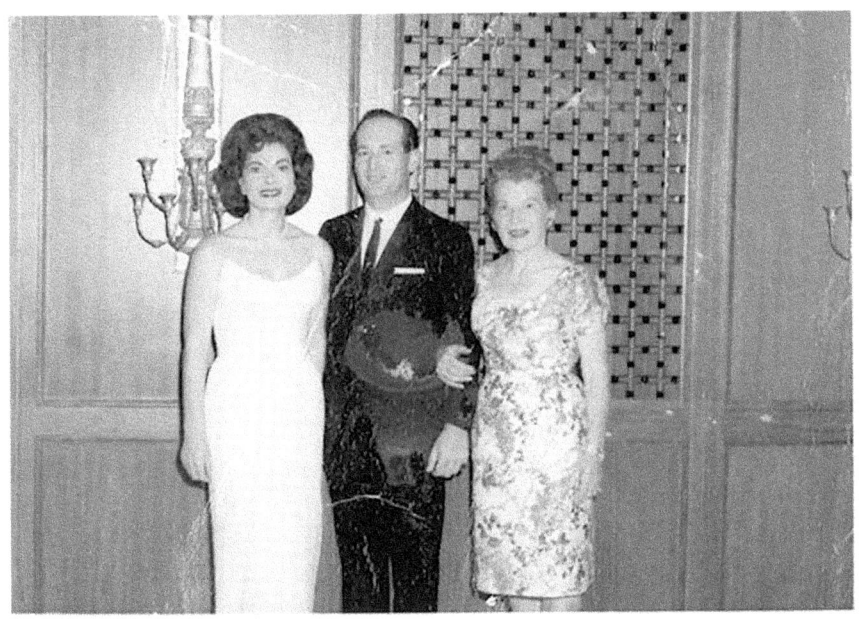

Harriett (my mother), Uncle Bob and Grandma Ida

www.ingramcontent.com/pod-product-compliance
Ingram Content Group UK Ltd.
Pitfield, Milton Keynes, MK11 3LW, UK
UKHW022226230426
12048UKWH00016BA/1084